Praise for Tami Brady's Books

"This book is a passionate, intense account of one person's conquest over suffering. As such, it will validate the experience of others struggling with Fibromyalgia and Chronic Fatigue Syndrome, inspire and empower them to make changes, and provides a template for them to follow. As a psychologist working with chronic pain sufferers, I can endorse Ms. Brady's philosophy, approach and tools."

—Bob Rich, PhD, author *Cancer: A Personal Challenge*

"The main point I saw in this work, and one I thought was outstanding, is that we are all individuals, unique and that one set formula may not work for everyone. I believe that is what makes her work different than other self-help books."

—Shirley Johnson, *Midwest Book Review*

"I found myself submersed in this book, discovering it a true source of encouragement, that however overwhelming life becomes, we should stay aware of what we want, never forgetting where we come from or what our dreams are."

—Tracy Jane-Newton, *An Alternative View*

"…a fresh alternative in a sea of self-help books. Brady shows how to break free of a debilitating prison of low self-esteem while strengthening the independent woman waiting to be released Her thought-provoking questions lead her readers to gain independence, confidence, and get their lives back on the road it was meant to take. Hope is within - and Brady has the keys."

—Vicki Landes, *Reader Views*

"I found it helpful for self-examination and analysis. The author helped me gain insights into my personal behavior patterns and in understanding myself in relation to the world around me. Tami Brady is a very articulate and an excellent communicator. The book is designed to help the reader discover for themselves an understanding of their own unique personality."

—Richard R. Blake

"The author is not a mental health professional: everything she writes about she has experienced first-hand. It is brimming with exercises and lists of useful resources, including an impressive array of online help and information websites. The author's advice emerges from a coherent philosophy of life and this lends the book pragmatic sagacity that many other, far heftier tomes, lack. Recommended."
—Sam Vaknin, PhD, author *Malignant Self Love: Narcissism Revisited*

"Brady's goal is to have the reader explore their true self. She goes on to call attention to our penchant to live by 'expectations that our not your own'. I appreciate Tami Brady's intent to help people discover their truth so that we all can live authentic lives. She presents ideas in an organized format and provides both background information and tools to incorporate new knowledge."
—Erika K. Oliver, *Reader Views*

"...A perfect and simple way to begin the process of transforming one's life and living the unique purpose that resides within the soul."
—Richard A. Singer Jr., MA, CAC, *Your Daily Walk with the Great Minds*

"If you have been thinking there must be more to life than what you have; or you find you tend to say one thing in public, whilst being of another opinion in private, then this book may be for you."
—Sue Phillips, *Spiralthreads Reviews*

"...One of the best guidebooks I have read and yet it does not overwhelm the reader with daunting tasks and unrealistic expectations."
—Angela Hutchinson, *Spirit-Works.Net*

"You can almost feel the warmth of her words radiate throughout your body as you allow each one to absorb deep into your soul. Allow her to come into your life and you will discover the person you were truly meant to be."
—Suzie Housley, *MyShelf.com*

Strategies:

A Chronic Fatigue Syndrome and Fibromyalgia Journey

TAMI BRADY

First printing March 2008

Library of Congress Cataloging-in-Publication Data

Brady, Tami, 1968-
Strategies : a chronic fatigue syndrome and fibromyalgia journey / Tami Brady.
    p. cm.
    ISBN-13: 978-1-932690-48-4 (trade paper : alk. paper)
    ISBN-10: 1-932690-48-4 (trade paper : alk. paper)
    1. Brady, Tami, 1968---Health. 2. Chronic fatigue syndrome--Patients--Biography. 3. Fibromyalgia--Patients--Biography. I. Title.
    RB150.F37B73 2008
    616'.0478--dc22

                                        2007050897

Distributed by: Baker & Taylor, Ingram Book Group, Quality Books
Loving Healing Press
5145 Pontiac Trail
Ann Arbor, MI 48105
USA

http://www.LovingHealing.com or
info@LovingHealing.com
Fax +1 734 663 6861

Loving Healing Press

Disclaimer

This publication is sold with the understanding that the publisher is not engaged in rendering medical treatment, health care, or other professional advice. If medical treatment is required, the services of a competent professional person should be sought. Before adding, removing, or changing any medication, therapy, or procedure it is your responsibility to notify and consult with your physician.

About our Series Editor, Robert Rich, Ph.D.

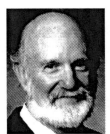

Robert Rich, M.Sc., Ph.D., M.A.P.S., A.A.S.H. is a highly experienced counseling psychologist. His web site www.anxietyanddepression-help.com is a storehouse of helpful information for people suffering from anxiety and depression.

Bob is also a multiple award-winning writer of both fiction and non-fiction, and a professional editor. His writing is displayed at www.bobswriting.com. You are advised not to visit him there unless you have the time to get lost for a while.

Three of his books are tools for psychological self-help: *Anger and Anxiety, Personally Speaking*, and *Cancer: A personal challenge*. However, his philosophy and psychological knowledge come through in all his writing, which is perhaps why three of his books have won international awards, and he has won many minor prizes. Dr. Rich currently resides at Wombat Hollow in Australia.

Books by Tami Brady

The Complete Being: Finding and Loving the Real You (2006)
Blame and Judgment (2006)
From Lost to Found (2006)
Regaining Control: When Love Becomes a Prison (2007)
Usui Reiki Ryoto: Level One (2007)
Usui Reiki Ryoto: Level Two (2007)
Strategies: A Chronic Fatigue Syndrome and Fibromyalgia Journey (2008)

Table of Contents

Preface

In the spring of 1997, I got what I thought was a really bad case of the flu. It wasn't. My symptoms worsened and after consultation with numerous specialists I was eventually diagnosed with Chronic Fatigue Syndrome and Fibromyalgia. I spent the next decade alternately denying my illness and trying to find a cure so I could get back to my regular life. Instead, what I found was an entirely different existence filled with countless strategies to deal with my symptoms.

In the years since, I have viewed my health conditions as both my downfall and the most amazing gift I have ever been given. My period of denial pushed me to do some really amazing things. I completed both my BA and MA in archaeology and heritage, with honours and distinction. I started my own archaeological consulting company. I wrote and published my first book, a self-help work titled *The Complete Being: Finding and Loving the Real You*. I created online courses, wrote several regular columns, served as contributor liaison for an archaeological magazine, and acted as dean for an online university.

My period of acceptance led me to a quieter place, where I have the ability to be myself without excuse or embarrassment; where my health and my family are my main priorities; where I feel loved and valuable for the person I am; where I feel free to undertake work that I feel is important and worthwhile; and where I am content.

Sometimes, on bad days, I feel isolated and depressed. I am angry that my life has been taken from me. It's a struggle to use what little energy and strength I have to get through the day. Thoughts of my lost dreams and the knowledge that tight budgets will always be my constant companions are sometimes almost too much to bear.

Still, these realizations and moments of darkness make me treasure my good days. On these brighter days, I feel like I am exactly where I need to be. Each experience, each page that gets written in a frenzy of activity, every time I don't huff and puff when I climb the hill behind my house, and whenever I remember some tiny bit of trivia that I had thought was forever forgotten in the "fibrofog" of the day before, I realize that I am blessed. I know how much of my life I had previously been taken for granted. I remember how little I actually listened to and enjoyed my children in the past. I see what's really truly important.

What follows is the story of my experiences: how I got to a more peaceful place and the struggles that I continue to work through each day. Those of you with Chronic Fatigue Syndrome and Fibromyalgia will likely see yourself in my experiences. Although our symptoms and our paths to find balance and contentment might differ, having these health issues impacts our life in ways that we could never have imagined even in our wildest dreams (or nightmares as the case may be). In the end, we are all changed forever. On good days, I believe for the better.

1 How It Started

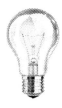

"All growth is a leap in the dark, a spontaneous unpremeditated act without the benefit of experience."
—Henry Miller (1891-1980)

The spring of 1997 was both a time of great hope and a period of great stress. I had been going through a number of major changes in my life. For about four years, I had been working at a local museum as a glorified tour guide. When I first started at the museum, I absolutely loved it. Before that point, I had been a stay-at-home-mom. Before that I was in high school. Despite the seeming hopelessness of my situation, I had always hoped to go to university and study archaeology and history. Working at the museum was my personal test to see if I really liked history enough to do it for a living. Secretly, I also wanted to be sure that I was smart enough to actually take in large amounts of academic information.

I started out at the museum as a volunteer and although I am a fairly introverted person, I blossomed as a tour guide. Before the first season was complete, I was asked to take a paid part-time position the following year.

I read every book I could get my hands on. I listened intently to my supervisor who was a wealth of information. It felt great to share my newfound knowledge with others and freeing to have amazing academic conversations with my colleagues. My self confidence rose to new heights until I actually believed I was smart enough to go to university and earn my degree.

In the summer of 1995, I started taking university level correspondence courses in history and anthropology with the intention of transferring over to the local university full time in the fall of 1997, when my youngest child started school full time. Although the course work was demanding, I fell into university study like I had been born for it. I was organized and managed to take care of my duties at home, at work, and still get good marks. I felt I was ready for more.

In 1996, the museum hired a new curator. This new curator wasn't a people person like the previous one. She micromanaged, was straight by the book, and brought with her a wave of political chaos that left everyone feeling undervalued and attacked. Staff members took sides, volunteers quit, and everyone was miserable. I eventually dreaded going to work. By the spring of 1997, I was more than ready to quit and start full time university classes.

At home, my life also started to fall apart. My father-in-law was preparing for open heart surgery. It was agreed that he and my mother-in-law would stay with us during the process. I don't think I had a clue what I was in for and I don't think I was really that realistic in my vision of what this surgery might entail.

I love my in-laws and even believe that they love me in their own way. However, we have never really gotten along. To this day, I'm not sure if it's because we are so very different (different lifestyles, values, belief systems, and life goals) or if it's because we are so very alike (all or nothing thinking, unable to share our true feelings, and most importantly a strong sense of family protectiveness). The truth is that I think I agreed to having my in-laws stay at our house just so that they would accept me into the family and love me the way I needed to be loved by them. I was so very naïve.

We soon found out that heart surgery isn't a one time event of a few weeks of stress. My father-in-law had almost a year of tests and consultations before the actual surgery. A few times a month, he and my mother-in-law would stay with us for a week or two for another round of tests or yet another set of appointments. We were all stressed, frustrated and scared. We all wanted to get the operation done and over before my father-in-law had another heart attack. No one talked about the "what ifs" but these unsaid thoughts took over every aspect of our lives. The surgery was eventually scheduled for the fall of 1997, just as I was entering university.

There was no doubt that I was under a lot of stress (from work, the worries about my father in-law, the financial stress of housing two extra people, and the anxiety over starting university in the fall), so it didn't really surprise me that I got a lot more colds during the winter of 1996-

97. It seemed like I would just get rid of one bout of flu and the next week I had a cold. I was getting pretty run down and bitchy but I persevered.

Later that spring, I had what I thought was a really bad case of the flu. My body was one big ache and the fatigue was debilitating. It knocked me flat on my back to a point where completing daily chores became almost impossible. This was definitely not a good situation when I already felt that my in-laws thought that I was a bad housekeeper and wife.

I eventually went to the local clinic to see if there was something I could do to get over this horrible flu bout. Regrettably, the appointment didn't go quite as I expected. The doctor told me that I could have glandular fever (a.k.a. mononucleosis) and took a blood test. Now, I was really upset. I was sure that the only way I could have contracted mononucleosis was if my husband was cheating on me. After all, in high school everyone called it "the kissing disease". I was pretty angry and it was a long week until the tests came back negative.

Unfortunately, even though the tests were negative for mononucleosis, my worries weren't yet over. The doctor told me that he had no idea why I was sick but that it was definitely something because my white cell count was irregular. I believe he told me to consult my family doctor but that's a little fuzzy in my memory.

The next few weeks were a blur of bad getting horribly worse. I was tired and depressed. I was so ready to quit my job that I could feel the bile rise every time I thought about the museum. At the time, I was leading a team of guys undertaking historical reconstruction of vertical log buildings. Basically, we carried logs, we cut logs, we dug trenches, we put the logs in the trench, and then we buried the bottoms of the logs. In good health, it was tough work (made particularly difficult by being the only woman on the crew and a good 75 lbs lighter than most of these construction-type guys). Although I had done this work the year before with few problems, I noticed that I got tired much more quickly this season. My aches and pains never seemed to go away. My back was always hurting. I was pretty miserable.

Then, one day I was planting a log in the trench and my legs gave way. Everyone thought I had just slipped but I knew something was very wrong. There had been a few times when my legs felt like lead and every step sent shooting pains up my legs. My vision had also been acting erratically. I could see perfectly fine one moment and then a fog would impede my vision for a few days.

I was beginning to become concerned and really quite frightened. My Dad's sister had just been diagnosed with Multiple Sclerosis. Many of the symptoms she described sounded just like my issues. I was terrified that I also had MS, so I made an appointment with my family doctor.

Let me say that I really don't like doctors. I've had a lot of bad experiences with them. When I was a child, I was severely hard of hearing. Although I was a regular at the doctor's office (a seemingly constant stream of colds and flu made worse by a myriad of different allergies), no one ever noticed that I had a hearing problem until it was brought to their attention by my kindergarten teacher, who noticed that I was adept at reading lips. When I was seven, they found the cure to my hearing difficulties, by accident during a tonsillectomy. Once my tonsils were taken out, I could suddenly hear perfectly. Evidentially, my adenoids were so large that my eardrums couldn't vibrate properly, causing the hearing loss.

When I was sixteen, I was diagnosed with endometriosis. This diagnosis took several years with countless doctors telling me that my pain was all in my head. Eventually, after I suffered from a cyst in my ovary, a specialist found the problem. Without any sort of gentle bedside manner, he abruptly told me that I would never have children. Not only did this news send me into a deep suicidal depression but he was wrong. I was blessed with three healthy naturally conceived children before I was 22 years old!

My final pregnancy was quite difficult. I started having contractions in my fifth month of pregnancy and we were all terrified that I would lose the baby. My family doctor somewhat callously told me that the longer my child stayed in the womb, the more likely it would survive. She gave no instructions for bed rest and no strategies about how to deal with severe cramps that lasted 4-8 hours every day. I ended up at the hospital several times sure that it was time to deliver the baby just to be sent home with a feeling that I was being silly. When my son eventually did arrive (5 days late), my labor pains weren't at all regular, and lasted an hour and a half total. We didn't even get a chance to get to the hospital so my husband caught our son as he entered this world.

After that pregnancy, I knew having any more children would be too risky. We had gotten lucky to get a healthy full term child but we knew that trying again would be pushing it. I made arrangements with a specialist to get my tubes tied and cauterized. He agreed to do the tube tying but felt that I was too young to make a rational decision on the cauterization. My grandmother had had several babies after her tubes were tied and failed so I was quite adamant on making sure that this procedure was permanent. This doctor tried bullying me and even tried sneakily setting up the procedure he wanted, but eventually I got what I wanted.

These experiences really negatively coloured my view of doctors. I thought that most medical practitioners were insensitive, arrogant and incompetent. I felt that if you had anything more than the common cold (take liquids and get some rest), that medical practitioners had no clue what to do to help you. Far too often, their reaction was that if they didn't know what to do it about a particular condition, it must somehow be in your head.

I have since realized that doctors are merely human. Just like the rest of us, they'd rather be golfing than giving us a pap test and pray for a quick easy day so that they can get home to friends and family. Who can blame them?

Despite my misgivings and past bad experiences, my family doctor at the time seemed quite competent and sincere. When we discovered that my second daughter had a strange lump on her chest, our doctor had been diligent. A CAT scan was arranged in no time and the lump was quickly diagnosed as a harmless lump of cartilage. Throughout the whole experience, my family doctor seemed to understand our concerns and was more than willing to help make sure that no harm would come to our child.

If any doctor could help me with my own health problems, I felt this one could. Besides, if I did have MS, I wanted to know sooner rather than later. At least that's what I thought at the time. In retrospect though, I'm not so sure I really wanted to know the truth. I definitely wasn't ready for it. How could I have possibly known that my life was about to change so very, very much?

2 The Doctor's Visit

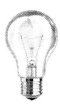

"Don't tell your problems to people: eighty percent don't care; and the other twenty percent are glad you have them."
—Lou Holtz (1937-)

The next year was an extended exercise in frustration and futility. By the time I got to my doctor's appointment my symptoms were rapidly getting worse. My legs hurt and were weak. My knees buckled regularly. Under regular circumstances, I don't sleep a lot. I tend to sleep best in the hours before midnight and don't get much rest after that point. Four or five hours of sleep is usually more than enough for me to survive but at this point I was rarely getting two good hours of sleep each night. My vision went wacky sometimes, often for a few days at a time. I was confused and kept getting my opposites (right and left, north and south, up and down, etc) mixed up.

My first visit to my family doctor went fairly smoothly, if not very genially. She gave me a lot of grief for not having had a regular examination for a few years and told me she was sure that my thyroid was the problem. Then my doctor went on an all out tirade, telling me that it was my fault that the condition worsened to such an extent because if I had regular checkups she would have found the thyroid condition before it caused all these problems. Now, given the severity of the situation, the medications might not bring me back to normal. At the time, I felt she was right to berate me because I was in the wrong so I took what bordered on abuse without any sort of resistance.

I was immediately sent for tests to check my thyroid and another appointment was made. It was expected that the doctor would give me medication and lay out the lifestyle changes that needed to be made at this next appointment. This was obviously not meant to be.

In the weeks that followed, my condition continued as it had. In the interim, I started school and my father-in-law finally had his surgery.

Actually, I started school the week that my father-in-law had his operation.

I loved school and did very well in the classes but there were several situations that were quite unbearable, especially at first. I had been brought up in a little town of under 10,000 people. Until, I was six, we had lived outside of town and I saw very few people who weren't relatives. During this time, our only trips into town were to the doctor every few months when I needed medical care. When I was six, we moved into town, which was a complete shock to my system and I became incredibly shy. To say the least, going to a university that had 40,000 people was a little much to take. For the first three weeks, it took every ounce of courage I had not to run home and hide. Fighting the fear of the crowds was absolutely exhausting.

The situation with my in-laws made matters worse. Tensions were high and my in-laws react quite differently to anxiety than I do. After his surgery, we went to visit my father in-law once a day for a short visit. I had been raised in a family where hospital visits started when visiting hours began and ended when the staff finally kicked you out each night. When the patient slept, the waiting room became a temporary refuge. Flowers and presents were brought to cheer up the room. At the time, I couldn't comprehend that my family's actions indicated love, compassion, and hopes that my father-in-law would take the time to rest. I also didn't realize that we all react differently to stressful situations. I thought that my mother-in-law was cold and that my husband was in complete denial.

By this time, I regularly walked with a cane (euphemistically named George) and my legs were like rubber most of the time. My temper was short. My generalized pain and fatigue were getting so bad that I could hardly function. Keeping my house clean to my mother-in-law's standards (which I had never managed to achieve with full health) was impossible. I felt like my in-laws treated me like I was faking my symptoms to get attention or because I was lazy. My husband was pretty distant, for obvious reasons, so I had no one on my side. I was pretty miserable.

The tone of my next doctor's appointment was slightly different. As you probably guessed, I didn't have a thyroid condition. I could tell that the doctor was completely at a loss. At the time, I thought she handled this pretty well. She began testing me for every conceivable illness or condition known to man. I had all sorts of blood tests and urine tests. I'm really not sure what these were all about but on the next visit she told me that she had ruled out chemical imbalances, vitamin deficiencies, accidental poisonings, cancer, diabetes, lupus, and a myriad of other complicated-sounding conditions.

The doctor admitted that she was stumped. It was then that I told her that I was concerned that I had Multiple Sclerosis. I told her about my aunt's history of the condition. My doctor listened and said that she thought that this might be a big possibility given my symptoms and the family history. She arranged for me to see a neurology specialist.

The waiting time for the consultation was six months.

During this time, my in-laws stayed at our house just as regularly as in the previous year. There were even more follow up checks and more doctors' appointments than there had been before the actual operation. My father-in-law also ended up in the hospital for his prostate. At this point, I was convinced that my in-laws hated me even more than they had before the surgery. I also realized that we were never going to be best buddies and they were never going to hug me and tell me that they were glad that their son married me. Every "visit" threatened to end my marriage as my husband and I fought horribly.

School became my refuge of sorts. I had made a few friends, my marks were good, and a few of the professors even knew my first name. I loved the energy and feeling of hope that resounded in the hallways and in the classrooms. My favourite place was the library. Here, I read every book I could get my hands on. I particularly loved writing papers because I got to spend weeks filling up my backpack with books that I read all night when I wasn't sleeping anyway. Although I was constantly in pain and the fatigue was often unbearable, for the first time in my life I felt like I was exactly where I should be.

The neurology specialist visit was quite trying to my patience. I took the day off school, which was frustrating. Despite all of my pain, fatigue, and having to tromp around the campus with my cane, I only missed three classes during my entire university career. This was something I took great pride in so I was very irritated when I had to miss any school at all.

My time in the waiting room at the neurologist's office actually took longer than the actual consultation. I waited for what seemed to be hours in the waiting room. Once I was in the office, the doctor quickly went over my history and my symptoms. He then did a few balance tests, some prick tests, and hit my knee with that little mallet (like in the movies). He was extremely aloof during the whole process and simply ignored my questions. At the end of the visit, he told me we'd do an MRI. I left his office feeling confused and wondering what had just happened. I had no clue what the MRI was for and wondered if the doctor felt that I could have MS or not.

More waiting. It took six weeks to get the MRI done. I had another appointment scheduled with my family doctor about three weeks after the MRI was complete. My family doctor hadn't gotten the diagnosis from the neurologist yet but the MRI showed ten white lesions on my brain. My doctor and the MRI technician were sure that this meant I did indeed have Multiple Sclerosis. Still, all we could was wait for the neurologist's official diagnosis.

This process took several more weeks and when I finally got the ruling I was at a loss. The doctor didn't state that I didn't have MS but simply said that at this point in time he wasn't willing to say that the lesions were indicative of MS. He'd need to create a history of changes in the MRI over a period of time (perhaps years) to make such a determination.

My family doctor decided that, in the meantime, we would go another route. I call this period the "you might be crazy" line of examination. I went to a generalist doctor who did more tests for cancer and lupus. He also asked me if my husband was abusing me and if I were sexually abused as a child. Basically, they wanted to check to see if I was manifesting some sort of post traumatic stress type illness. Sorry, I'm pretty boring and apart from living with imaginary pain and fatigue for nine months, I'm pretty stable thank you very much.

I also had a full psychological evaluation. It was like out of some weird movie: someone sitting behind the glass taking notes, a camera recording my every expression, and several doctors in white lab coats and carrying clipboards playing good doctor bad doctor. Tell me about your relationship with your mother. Does your husband abuse you? Did someone ever touch you wrong? I spent the entire session feeling like at any moment someone was going to show up, wrestle me to the ground, put a straight-jacket on me, and take me away to the loony bin.

Fortunately, that didn't happen. They sent me on my way, simply saying that I was stressed out and they'd send their report to my family doctor within ten days. Two weeks later, she still hadn't gotten the diagnosis.

The actual diagnosis was that I was a perfectionist who pushed herself too hard. I could have told you that. Hell, anyone that's ever met me could tell you that. But it didn't explain why I had to walk with a cane, why I hurt so much, why I felt confused most of the time, why I couldn't sleep, and why I could hardly get out of bed each morning. The only bright spot in my life at the time was that school was out for the summer session so I was again a stay-at-home-mom for a couple of months.

Since the neurological diagnosis, or lack thereof, the thought of endless consultations and no relief in sight had started to get me down. At my next appointment, I told my doctor I was extremely frustrated. I was slightly taken aback when her demur suddenly changed to utter joy. She started asking me if I felt I was depressed, if my sadness affected the rest of my life, and if I ever thought about suicide. This was an extremely stupid line of questioning in my mind. When you are in pain all the time, it goes without saying that you feel blue and are discouraged. It makes sense that that this feeling permeates through your every thought. Who, in all honesty, wouldn't think once in a while that ending it all wasn't the answer?

But my doctor got the answer she wanted to make her feel in charge again. I was depressed! Now, she could prescribe something! She gave me sleeping pills and antidepressants. I would take the sleeping pills every night whether I needed them or not and the antidepressants for a minimum of nine months.

It was decided that we'd also try one more specialist and then wait six months or so for another neurology exam. This particular specialist was a sports medicine professional. I really didn't hold much hope for this appointment so another month of waiting didn't really faze me. Plus, I was pretty doped up during that time. To tell you the truth, I don't remember much from that period. I slept a lot. I moved only to check on the kids and make supper. My house was a mess and the laundry was never done.

I was a extremely bitter person. I knew I had MS and was pissed off that I would have to wait for the diagnosis.

I knew that I would have to take at least a year off of school. With the pills I was taking, I couldn't take care of myself each day let alone keep up with school work. This thought nearly crushed me. I knew if I took a year off, I wasn't ever going back to school. I knew that my symptoms were getting progressively worse and a wheelchair was in my immediate future.

During this time, I was a completely inept mother. Up to this point, I had been a really hands on Mommy. I made bunny shaped cakes for Easter, created special activities booklets for each of my three kids, knew all their friends' names, and regularly took them for excursions to the bird sanctuary or to feed the geese at the park. Now, my kids were pretty much taking care of themselves. If some sort of emergency had happened, I truly don't know if I could have even called an ambulance.

After only a few weeks of living in a foggy world of drugs, I decided that I wanted my life back. I made an appointment with my doctor and told her that I wasn't going to take the pills anymore. In my mind, a life of pain, fatigue, and depression was preferable to endangering my children's lives by not really being there to take care of them.

My family doctor washed her hands of me.

I waited for the final specialist appointment.

In the meantime, I started reading up on Multiple Sclerosis, pain and fatigue. I started looking into vitamins, herbals supplements and Chinese medicines. I set myself up a system of a combination of these three traditions. Basically, it was a combination of anti-oxidant treatment and everything I could find for fatigue. This included flax seed oil, vitamin E, some B vitamins, poria, magnolia, and a lot of Bee Pollen. I also read a lot of books on meditation and began a strict routine of meditation for stress relief and pain management.

By the time I got my appointment for the sports medicine specialist, I was feeling slightly better. I was still dragging my butt, I still wasn't getting much sleep, and my body still hurt but I felt that I had some aspect of control of my own destiny once again. I felt that through my own efforts, I could survive and get back to living my life to some extent. Once in a while, I even managed to exercise a bit.

What should have been the climax of my experience went surprisingly fast, smooth, and with few dramatics. I waited perhaps fifteen minutes in the waiting room at the sports medicine specialist's office and then was called into the examination room. My husband didn't go in with me to this particular examination as he had previously done with most of my other appointments. We naturally assumed that there would be several more consultations before I got any sort of diagnosis.

Once in the examination room, the doctor asked me about my pain and fatigue: same old, same old. Then, she started touching different points on my body. A good many of these points were excruciatingly painful but a few actually felt good. I remember a chart on the wall illustrating the exact points that she was touching. I also recall that she was very gentle and actually listened to my answers when she asked me questions. The specialist also explained what she was doing as she was doing it.

Before the specialist was completely done with the examination, she was already explaining to me that I had Fibromyalgia and that she had been testing trigger points. Pain and irritation in a majority of these trigger points in association with my symptoms, and the lack of another answer, indicated Fibromyalgia. She also said that the fatigue was caused by Chronic Fatigue Syndrome which often coupled with Fibromyalgia. Finally, she told me that having these conditions wouldn't kill me but it could make my life a living hell.

When I asked what I could do to help the condition, the specialist told me that there was no cure and no medications that would actually get rid of these conditions. Yes, my family doctor could put me back on antidepressants and sleeping pills but they would only mask the situation. When I showed her my list of vitamins, herbs, Chinese medicines, she said that they wouldn't hurt me and if I felt some relief by taking them to keep it up. She said exercise, even if it caused a lot of pain, would help. She also encouraged me to keep up with my meditation.

No follow up visits. No care regime. The rest was left up to me.

Finally, I had my answer. I decided that future visits with my family doctor would be an exercise in futility. I was doing more for myself and my care than my doctor had done in a year. In fact, I've only gone back to my family doctor once since I was diagnosed with Chronic Fatigue Syndrome and Fibromyalgia, when I thought that I'd had a heart attack. The doctor frantically tested me, making me believe I had a heart condition and left me with the advice that I should lose a few pounds, take calcium supplements, and have regular check ups.

A few months before I started writing this book, I found out on a discussion group that these chest pains are common with those that suffer from Fibromyalgia and are nothing to worry about. In fact, when you believe that you are having a heart attack, you often end up having a panic attack, which makes the situation that much more scary. The best explanation I've heard about these chest pains is that the neurons in the brain become overloaded and fire randomly until the body resets itself naturally. Once it does, the pain will end. Actually, that sounds like a pretty apt description of the majority of my pain symptoms.

3 Denial – Part I

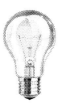

"Fuck it. Let's do it."

—Australian Proverb

Denial can get you through a lot and I spent almost a decade in deep, deep denial. This was a crazy period of my life. To this day, I'm not sure how I survived. I do know that I was driven, insanely and unhealthily to do so.

I left the sports medicine specialist with a strange sense of calm. I had read in one of the many books that some patients with Fibromyalgia sometimes get Multiple Sclerosis in later years. This diagnosis seemed to give credence to my belief that I had MS. At the time, I really thought that Fibromyalgia and Chronic Fatigue Syndrome were made up illnesses to gently help a person deal with the fact that they had MS.

I was sure that my life was over. I could see myself in a wheelchair. I could see myself being unable to take care of myself let alone live a happy life. I could see all my hopes and dreams disappearing.

Instead of wallowing in my despair, something miraculous happened. I was told by the university board that I could definitely take a year off school but that I would have to start repaying on my student loans right away. I had no extra income at the time as I had quit my job at the museum the summer before I started university, believing it to be the sole cause of my stress. We couldn't afford to repay the loans I owed so I decided I needed to stay in school.

At the same time, I came upon the stark realization that few people who studied archaeology actually became archaeologists. Most archaeology majors became secretaries. I learned that only those students that could get into graduate school actually had a small chance at getting employment after graduation. By holding a Master's degree and illustrating that they have the appropriate amount of archaeological practical experience, these few individuals gained the unique ability to hold an archaeological permit, which made them employable as crew chiefs and project managers. To get into graduate school, my GPA had to be 3.30 (out of 4.0) or higher, I had to have excellent references, I had to be published, and I had to undertake an honours thesis that was professional in research, writing, and content.

I became manically driven like I had been given a death sentence. I became fixated on getting into graduate school. I did reduce my course load as much as I could to compensate for my "illness", but I also took night classes and summer classes to make up this lost time. I worked my school schedule around my family. I was always home when my children left each morning for school and was usually back before them. I used my insomnia as quiet study time and long bus rides to read even more books to get an edge over my fellow students. I even baked bread for some crazy reason to prove I was super human. I could be everything to everyone. I wasn't lazy, or crazy, and I definitely wasn't going to fail!

I read more. I studied harder. I slept less. I meditated more. I drank Bee Pollen like it was candy. Believe me that really was really quite a feat because frankly the stuff tastes like feet. Please excuse the bad pun. You don't want to know what's really in it though, believe me.

I began changing in those next few years. I refused to use my cane, even when I could hardly hold myself upright. No one at school knew I was sick. Despite this fact, most students thought I was superwoman by merely being an honours student, doing extra research on the side, and taking care of a family. If they'd only known the truth, they would have called up the loony bin.

At home, the subject of my health was taboo. Although my family sometimes caught me limping or cringing, we never openly mentioned my pain or noted my fatigue. Yes, my symptoms were reduced and not as debilitating (probably a constant 7 rather than the 9.75 out of ten that I had been experiencing) but they hadn't gone away. I simply trained myself that if I hurt more then I worked even harder to distract myself. If I was going to be disabled and have a shortened life, as I believed, I was going to get as much as I could done before that happened.

I tried to ignore the situation but a couple of unfortunate incidents reminded me of the truth. My most traumatic episode occurred while I was at archaeological field school. For about a month and a half, I was one of about twenty students housed in cabins near our archaeological site.

Every morning, we hiked several miles up the side of a mountain to the site with our equipment on our backs. Every evening, we hiked back down and spent the rest of night trying to get sand out of our ears, sharing stories about which part of our bodies hurt the most, and discussing the best lines of our favourite Monty Python movies. There was also a little partying and some great food prepared by one of my fellow students who I think missed his calling as a chief.

The actual site was spectacular. We were digging on a sandy beach (hence all the sand in our ears). There was a huge water reservoir to one side of the site and dense forest to the other. On all sides of us were beautiful mountains dipped in snow. Mountain sheep often stood on the ridge just mere meters from us. At lunch, we sat on huge glacial rocks that could fit four or five of us, and watched the waves roll in.

Not to get too technical, but the archaeological work was just as amazing. The findings were landmark. One of my colleagues found a Plainview point, which is extremely rare, one of the oldest finds in Western Canada. Another student found a skull from an archaic form of bison, which was also uncommon. It was truly an honour just to dig at such an amazing excavation.

I'll admit I am extremely competitive. When our instructor said that real archaeologists dug three levels of earth per day, I took it as a personal challenge. When I saw that the guy beside me (the excellent chief guy who was also one of the best diggers on site) and the guy who had found the Plainview point on the other side of me (probably the fastest and most diligent digger I've ever met) had also taken up the challenge, I saw a competition. I pushed hard. Some days, I could hardly walk out of the site at night.

Then, the worst day of my life occurred. It was a Thursday. I was down in the hole. It was so deep that when I stood up, I could hardly see the surface. I normally dig standing up and kind of hunched over. This pose reduces the likelihood of disturbing the soil and possible artifacts beneath me as I am frantically trying to work. I was busy digging when suddenly both my legs gave way and I dropped unceremoniously into the dirt. I didn't want anyone to know what had just happened. I secretly hoped that my legs would magically get strong enough so I could get out of the pit by lunch. So I sat there and just dug.

Fortuitously, we had a screen goddess that day, one of my roommates. A screen god or goddess is a person whose job for the day is to screen all the dirt that we are digging up in case we miss a tiny bone or piece of stone when we are excavating. Usually, we have to do this process ourselves, which dramatically slows our progress because we have to climb out of the pit, screen our dirt, and then climb back down to continue digging. This can become quite a hassle as the excavation pit becomes deeper and deeper. So when someone volunteers for the job of screening, we are all extremely grateful, hence the god or goddess term.

The weather was extremely bitter that day. It rained, it sleeted, it hailed, and the wind pushed sand into the units faster than we could dig it out. We could hardly breathe. The excavation site kind of looked like an odd game of whack a mole. Every so often, a head would pop out a hole and they'd turn away from the wind, trying to catch a breath or two of fresh air. Then, just as suddenly, they'd pop back down to retrieve all the sand that was pouring into their work area. It really was an exercise in futility.

I defiantly sat in the sand and tried to keep digging. A few people noticed my misery and I even have a picture that someone took. They thought that it illustrated how bad the conditions could get and how truly miserable that archaeology can be. Little did they know...

My plan worked fine until I had to go to the bathroom. We had a flag system up on the hill past the big glacial rocks in the dense forest. If the flag was up, someone was using the bush. An alternate washroom area was about 500 meters up the beach behind some huge rocks.

I decided that the beach alternative was my best bet but I would definitely need help. I had my cane neatly tucked into my backpack in case this eventuality should ever happen but since both legs had collapsed, I would need someone to hold onto the other side of me to keep me upright. I also needed help getting out of the excavation pit. I quietly told the screen goddess that I needed help and we attempted to be as invisible as possible.

It didn't work. Getting me out of the hole, using just my arms was pretty distracting. By the time we started walking up the beach, everyone was watching us. I was completely embarrassed and knew that my secret was out. I could feel my archaeological career falling apart.

The instructor met me at my work station when I got back from my bathroom trip. I told her what was happening and only through sheer stubbornness and a lot of arguing did she let me go back to work. To this day, I have no idea why I thought that that would solve the problem or why I believed that my legs would suddenly get better before quitting time. Still, I got back in the hole and I dug. I was bent on proving that I was healthy, despite that obviously I wasn't. I was manic.

I dug until lunch time. With help, I got out of the pit and waited for the barrage of questions and pitying looks. I think it was quite a shock to most of my fellow classmates because they had never had any indications that I was in any way disabled or ill.

Chronic Fatigue Syndrome and Fibromyalgia are like that. No one sees scars or disfigurement so it's a shock to most people that you actually have something really wrong with you. That we become incredible actors to mask and hide the symptoms makes the situation that much more difficult. It's amazing how strong denial can be and what our minds will allow us to do to hide from the truth. It is not at all healthy or productive, but amazing none the less.

The instructor knew how stubborn I was and knew I would go back to work after lunch despite that every other student wanted to call it a day because of the horrible weather conditions. She ingeniously decided that we'd have an impromptu lecture huddled against the huge rocks. After the lecture was over, a boat arrived to transport me back to where our vehicles were located. I was unequivocally told that I was getting on that boat, even if I had to be carried (which I was). One of my roommates volunteered to go with me (truth is, she just wanted to avoid the long walk out of the site and enjoy the cool boat ride).

On my way to the boat, one of the students said something that has stuck with me to this day. I was telling him that I was completely humiliated. He simply said that I had nothing to be embarrassed for, that now everyone knew that I was human just like them. It was years before the full meaning of that statement would really set in.

I called my husband when I got back to the cabin and went home early for the weekend. I rested and my legs gained enough strength to walk again. Monday morning I was back at work. I do think I lost something in my instructor's eyes though. Before the incident, she had been asking me about my plans for graduate school. She was normally a project manager with a local consulting firm and she had indicated that she would give me a good reference so that I could get a job with them when I finished school.

After that day, she looked at me with veiled pity. I got demoted to washing artifacts and being screen goddess for a week. I was so embarrassed over "the incident" that once I finished school I applied to every other firm but my former instructor's. I didn't want anyone to know what could happen because I knew it meant the end of my career before it even got a chance to start. No one in their right mind would take on a disabled archaeologist. Archaeologists spend way to much time in the bush and in situations that are dangerous enough for completely healthy individuals. Getting a rescue for an injured worker is just plain expensive and with tight budgets and schedules being the norm in most archaeological projects, no one would ever chance such a possibility.

Over the next few years, I tried to forget that day and worked even harder to prove I was superhuman. Still, I never quite got over the fear that someone would find out about my flaws or that such an situation would occur again. I did manage to complete my undergraduate degree with all of the necessities needed to get accepted to graduate school. I also completed my MA with distinction while working for one of the professors, processing artifacts, conducting soil testing, and supervising his laboratory.

Despite that the pay was extremely poor, it was probably the best job I've ever had in my archaeological career. Every day I felt like I learned something new and I knew that I was making a difference. The professor was always open to new ways to process or look at the data and always willing to impart his extensive knowledge. I also had some of the deepest most profound conversations of my life in that dingy lab.

4   Denial – Part II

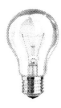

"Without fear and illness, I could never have accomplished all I have."

—Edvard Munch (1863-1944)

I completed my dissertation in the fall of 2002 and officially received my Master's degree in January of 2003. Archaeology season tends to taper off to almost nothing in the winter. Even those with MAs and years of experience can't find a job during that time of the year. I looked for a job but knew that I'd have to wait until May or June before I found anything solid so I continued working at the lab.

During my second year of graduate school, I had begun making extra money as a freelance writer. I mostly wrote articles but also ghostwrote a handful of e-books and did some "hire a cheat" term paper writing. That winter, I increased my writing activities to compensate for the low pay I was making at the lab.

What I didn't realize at that time was that archaeological work is synonymous with low paying jobs. Even during my first few archaeological jobs, I kept working at the lab in my off hours and then wrote at night to make a few bucks here and there.

To make matters worse, there is absolutely no security with archaeological jobs. Archaeologists are generally hired for one or two projects. They work as hard as they can until the work is done and then look for other work. It's pretty hard on the psyche, especially at first when you just can't understand why the company didn't give you more work and question whether you just weren't up to snuff. Truthfully, unskilled volunteers are lined up to do our job so we are reserved for situations where specialized training is essential.

In the fall of 2003, I thought I had finally made it. The government had granted my application for permit holding status so I could now become a crew chief or project manager. I got a job with a large international engineering firm. I was naïve so I thought that I my career was set and I had finally beaten the odds.

Life doesn't work that way for anyone. Plus, wasn't I forgetting something? Perhaps, a little think like Chronic Fatigue Syndrome and Fibromyalgia.

The truth is, I had almost myself convinced that I had been cured. I had pretty much given up the worry that I had Multiple Sclerosis, at least on the conscious level. I agreed with the sports medicine doctor that my symptoms had indeed been caused by Chronic Fatigue Syndrome and Fibromyalgia or "burn out" in my mind. I had long given up my regimen of vitamins, herbs and Chinese medicines. The only thing I had held onto was the meditation. With my job, I was getting lots of exercise and fresh air. I thought I was set.

I rarely got the debilitating fatigue anymore. For the most part, my symptoms were limited to pain in my back and legs and mental confusion (what I later learned was called fibrofog). Since I was working long hours and doing back-breaking work in difficult weather conditions, my aches, pains, and mental confusion seemed no different from anyone else's on the crew.

I was deep in denial. I truly believed I had cured myself. Hell, I even thought about writing a book about my experience and how I stomped out the disease. When I had symptoms, I blamed the fact that I had gained weight. "Once I lose a few pounds, I won't be putting so much pressure on my legs and they won't hurt. Of course, I'm tired with all this extra weight I have to work twice as hard as everyone else just to push this extra 45 lbs around."

I am so stubborn that the universe had to smack me on the head, and I still didn't quite get the message right away. I was on a fairly long term excavation where we were housed in motel rooms for about a month and a half. We got up every morning, dug all day, ate, went back to our motel rooms and slept. I popped extra strength Advil like candies, soaked in Epson salts until my skin looked like a raisin, went through countless tubes of A535, and had a Magic Bag (thermotherapeutic pack) collection to get me through the night so I could work the next day. Anyone really watching me would have thought I was a bit of a religious nut because I meditated every chance I could.

Still, once again, I had competition and was eager to prove myself. The first few weeks of the excavation, I was the top digger every single day. I even out-distanced everyone when I had to slow down my progress to intricately map out important features like cooking pits, hearths, pottery scatters, and patches of ochre that I was uncovering.

I was untouchable until a new crew member joined the excavation. It didn't matter to me that it had been weeks since I'd had a day off and this guy was fresh and eager to dig. Plus, this guy was a machine. Even at my top speed, I didn't have a chance at keeping up with him. That really irked me so I pushed harder. If my back ached, I just worked harder to distract myself.

One day, the pain became too much. I was nauseous and could hardly eat anymore. I had to sit down. I told my boss that I had messed my back up, which wasn't a complete lie. Given the type of work I was doing, back pain is a pretty common thing so I was told to rest until lunch and eventually (because I couldn't sit still) was told to do profiling, drawing pictures of the layers of dirt in the excavation pit.

That night, I got my boss to buy me a can of chicken noodle soup and I stayed at my motel room while everyone else went out for supper. I assured him that I didn't need to go to the hospital and that I just needed a little rest. That night, I called my husband and told him to come and get me but by the end of the conversation (after a good cry), I decided I couldn't go home.

I took the rest of the excavation a little slower. I slowed my pace from super archaeologist to somewhat normal human being. Okay, that's not entirely true but I did make an effort. I volunteered to profile more often that I really wanted. It just about drove me mad but I made it through the excavation and we went home.

I was glad that, soon after the excavation was complete, the workload slowed for the winter season. I was almost happy for the rest when I got called less and less often over the next few months. Well, almost.

5 Denial – Part III

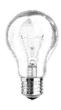

"Reality is merely an illusion, albeit a very persistent one."
—Albert Einstein (1879-1955)

Archaeology can be a very callous business. Usually, the only way that you know that you aren't going to be working for a particular company any longer is that you call and call and no more work comes your way. This was how I left my dream job. Apparently, there was no more work for me but no one told me straight out that I was no longer needed. No explanations. No pink slip. Eventually, I realized on my own that I'd have to find work elsewhere.

Overall, professionally speaking, I was in a really good position. I now had experience working on and leading over a dozen different archaeological jobs, ranging from a variety of survey projects and small urban residential projects to some substantial sized utilities and transportation projects. I had also held my own archaeological permits which gave me a good shot at any archaeological job that I wanted.

Then, fate stepped in. I thought it was the opportunity of a lifetime. I thought it was the answer to all my hopes and dreams. Perhaps, in a strange way it was.

While I was still hoping to get work from my dream company, early in 2004, I was given an opportunity to do an independent archaeological contract for another firm. Taking this project would allow me to get into archaeology for the oil and gas industry, which was just starting to take off. Moreover, doing the project would net me a substantial amount of money (a month's wages for a few days' worth of work).

I was eager to expand my resume and the prospect of "good" money was tempting, so I quickly jumped at the chance. I soon found that I really liked being my own boss and I loved working at home. I liked the ability to work at 2:00 am when I had insomnia, to get a few dishes done while waiting for return emails, and best of all to be home when the kids got back from school. While working as a "real" archaeologist, I had really lost track of my kids. They had come home from school to an empty house and basically policed themselves. Supper was usually courtesy of MacDonald's or Pizza Hut. I was feeling more and more disconnected (and guilty for choosing work over family) as time went on, but not bringing in an income really didn't seem like an option.

Doing independent contracts was the best of both worlds. I could earn good money and I could still keep the family connection intact. In time, I would also admit to myself and my family that working at home allowed me to take a little better care of my health and live more comfortably within my physical limitations.

I was fortunate. One contract turned into several. Eventually I made it legal and started my own archaeological contract firm, TCM. TCM was so named after the members of my family. Myself, my husband, and my kids (and even the cats strangely enough) all start with T, C, or M.

I became a subcontractor to several larger archaeological firms and took on a few projects every month, mostly in the oil and gas industry. It was a pretty great time. I would get assigned a project, jump in the truck, travel for a few hours, take a nice hike in some beautiful location, take a few pictures, and head back home. For the first while, I was completely taken aback that people would actually pay me good money to travel and go hiking.

I soon found out that contract work has its downside too. Like regular archaeological work, contracts are also feast or famine. I could have four contracts one week and then not see work for months. Tracking down payment for these contracts was often quite a feat in and of itself, often taking three to six months. The not knowing if I'd get paid and when I'd secure my next contract was somewhat difficult at times.

There was also another important factor. I freely admit that I am a workaholic and I thrive on adrenaline. I was never happier than when I had a bunch of contracts and very little time to complete them. I still think fondly of 20 hour work days and those unrealistic deadlines that I placed upon myself.

Since I feel most alive when I'm busy to distraction, being underemployed for long periods of time was extremely trying for me. I simply don't relax and I find it really hard to do anything just for the fun of it. I like purpose, working toward a goal, and getting things done.

I turned back to writing to fill up my spare time. I reviewed books for fun. I did some freelance work—articles and some more e-books. I also started to write courses for an online university. Eventually, I started writing a few regular columns for them as well, which led to low paying positions as Dean of Spirituality and Religion and Community Manager of History. These activities didn't earn a lot of money but they kept me somewhat sane. I felt like I had it all.

Still, when I had been in school and when I first started working in archaeology, I had always believed that the real reason my body hurt, my brain froze, and I got extremely tired was because I simply pushed myself too hard. Working at home allowed me the unique ability to take a closer look at my health. When I had insomnia, I could work to make up for those little naps that got me through my worst fatigue and pain bouts. I could meditate regularly. I didn't have to worry that colleagues might see me falter when I walked or that I had to recheck my written work to make sure I didn't mix up opposites. My writing even allowed me an outlet for my more spiritual and academic selves. It was quite a freeing experience.

Despite my new freedom though, my symptoms never completely disappeared. I still hurt a good deal of the time, particularly in my hips, legs, and back. Sometimes after a day of surveying, I could hardly hold myself up. Warm Epson salt baths, heating pads, and rest did little to help. I had almost constant headaches and random periods of fibrofog that often made thinking straight quite a challenge.

6 The Reality Check

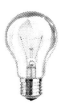

"I have had just about all I can take of myself."
—Samule N. Behrman (1883-1973)

The summer of 2005 was truly the pinnacle of my life. If my life would have ended that summer, it would have made a truly inspiring story: young girl from a small town overcomes many obstacles and fulfils her every dream. I had pretty much worked throughout the entire winter with various archaeological contracts and the spring had been just as busy. Despite being so busy with archaeological projects, I had written and self published my first e-book, The Complete Being.

Within a few weeks of publication of my e-book, I had lots of interest from magazines and radio shows wanting to interview me. Like I said, my life to that point made a pretty good story—even though I hadn't yet admitted to anyone that I had Chronic Fatigue Syndrome and Fibromyalgia. To top off my euphoria, Loving Healing Press contacted me, wanting to publish a print version of my book. I quickly agreed, signed the contract, and the book was published as *The Complete Being: Finding and Loving the Real You* in the spring of 2006.

I believe that the freedom I started to experience while working at home and writing that first book started to change me in ways I never thought possible. Much of what I did every day as a contract archaeologist and while writing that first book was about goal setting, working toward a particular dream, and focusing on the task at hand.

I was a master at these things. Despite my health issues, through goal setting, hard work and perseverance, I had achieved all that I had ever wanted. I had earned my degrees, gotten permit status, worked as a successful archaeologist, written a book, and still had time for my family. Wasn't I wonderful?

Yet, there was something somewhat hypocritical in my words and in the life I led. Something seemed a little forced perhaps. Most definitely, there were a few things about myself that I neither loved nor felt completely at peace with.

One of the underlying concepts of my book was that being genuinely yourself and finding personal truth would lead to a contented life. I had truly thought that I had been following my heart and living my dreams by becoming an archaeologist, but I started to think that being genuinely yourself had to do with something deeper, more profound. This was something I had missed somewhere along the way.

Yes, I love being an archaeologist. It's nice to go to a function where you can say you are an archaeologist when asked about your profession. Everyone knows what an archaeologist does and immediately shows a little more respect. Usually, they start to discuss their favourite discovery episode. It's a great icebreaker.

I also love the idea of archaeology. This is the romantic idea of finding lost civilizations, uncovering truths, and learning new things about the past. How very exciting, adventurous, and noble. I even like the realistic part of archaeology: travelling the countryside in an old beat up truck, eating burgers at diners, sleeping in motels in small towns, and walking for hours while surveying.

What's the problem, you ask? As an archaeologist, I had to pretend a lot: pretend that I didn't have Chronic Fatigue Syndrome and Fibromyalgia; pretend that I wasn't in pain or feeling tired; pretend that I wasn't worried that my legs might fall out from under me again; pretend that I was perfect and without any human flaws.

Somewhere along the way, the dream turned into a half truth and I began to feel like I was wearing a mask to hide my true identity. I was a fake. It was then that I realized that I had to find out who I really was and what dreams I truly wanted to cultivate. Ultimately, I realized that my goal in life wasn't to succeed at my career in some materialistic way, but it was to learn to love myself for all I've been and all that I am. This isn't an easy task.

Still, no sooner than had that realization started to wash over me, that destiny took over once again.

During that fall of 2005, there was a gradual wane in archaeological projects. At first, there was a bit of a lull. Then, there was a smattering of a few projects here and there. Finally, the work all but dried up.

In between projects, I had been spending a good deal of time and energy working for the online university. However, just as the archaeological work was beginning to dry up, the university made some major changes. I stopped writing my columns and gave up my positions as Dean and Community Manager. Only my courses stayed intact.

To say the least, I was pretty taken aback. I suddenly had my most secret wish. I had all the time in the world to "find myself". I could do anything I wanted. There was no one waiting to judge me or find out my secrets. I was free... how absolutely terrifying!

7   Transitions

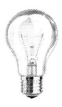

"We tend to forget that happiness doesn't come as a result of getting something we don't have, but rather of recognizing and appreciating what we do have."
—Frederick Koenig (1774-1833)

Of all the evolutions of my health condition so far, I think that this next phase was probably the hardest to bear. Strange, I wasn't in as much pain as in the first year of my diagnosis and I didn't have to push myself as hard as when I'd been in university. In fact, this part of my life was probably the most peaceful, free feeling, and unconditionally loving time that I've ever experienced. Yet, it was this part of my life that threatened to put me under. The best way I can describe this period was as grief. I think it took time and a lot of emotional energy to let go of all of those hopes, dreams, and fantasies that fell by the wayside in order to figure out what I really needed to do to live a happy, healthy, and contented life.

Fortunately, as often happens, when one opportunity is lost, another takes its place. One of my steady hobbies throughout the last few years had been reading and reviewing books. I love reading and learning new things, but with a tight budget books were a luxury I couldn't really afford. Getting free books in return for my opinion seemed the perfect answer so I started reviewing for several different online and print media. I enjoyed the process. Soon, I a lot of authors and publicists began contacting me directly for reviews of their books.

Somehow, I got it in my head to start my own review site, TCM Reviews. To my delight, the site was immediately successful. Within a month, I began to bring together an international team of reviewers. Review requests came pouring in and haven't stopped since we've opened our doors.

To keep up with the review requests and to build up the website, I reviewed a lot of self help literature, spiritual material, and books about health concerns. I tried to use what I learned in these resources to discover myself, try to find the missing pieces of my life, and most importantly figure out how to love myself unconditionally. I meditated, took long walks, kept a journal, and wrote poetry. I even wrote a short-lived blog about finding the genuine self, to force myself to focus on this path.

It was during this time period that I actually had my first strange twinges of something that I had never felt before: contentment. This experience was a complete revelation, enlightenment so to speak. I knew that in my life I had felt happy moments: the birth of my children, loving moments with my husband, fun family times, and some pride after successfully accomplishing a goal. However, as soon as something inevitably went wrong, the moment always seemed to fade and the good feelings quickly went away. Sometimes, I found that I couldn't even fully enjoy happy times because I knew that something bad would soon follow.

Contentment was something completely different. It felt like peace, like sunshine beaming down upon me on a warm summer day, the smile of a child, being in the loving arms of a parent, and like unconditional love. When I felt content, I knew I was in exactly the right place and doing just the right thing with my life no matter what chaotic mess or problems surrounded me. In those short moments, I was good enough, I earned enough money, I was healthy enough, and I had more than enough people to love me in just the right way. I had everything I needed right here and now.

I believe these small twinges gave me the strength and the courage to look deeper within myself for the answers. I began consciously gathering some insight into myself. I knew I was a workaholic and addicted to achieving. So long as I kept busy, I never had to deal with myself. I didn't have to acknowledge the pain that I was feeling (physically and mentally) and I didn't have to make peace with all those parts of myself that weren't perfect in my eyes.

At the time, I felt that the crux of my imperfections was the Chronic Fatigue Syndrome and Fibromyalgia. With these conditions, I would never be flawless. I would never be good enough. There would always be the worry that someone would find out that I was sick. There would always be the fear that my legs might give out or I might get too tired and have to rest. I might have to use my cane again. People would stare. Worse yet, people would give me that pitying look. Of all the pain and suffering that I have experienced in my life, that look easily has to be the most painful. It is almost lethal. In a single instant, I am brought down to nothing. I am broken and flawed. I am disabled.

At the time, the sheer overwhelming thought of dealing with my health issues was far too scary. Admitting that I had Chronic Fatigue Syndrome and Fibromyalgia would somehow make these illnesses real and permanent. I felt it would be like giving up and letting the conditions win. Ignoring the situation, however ridiculous (and no matter how clear it was that that wasn't working), seemed to be my only course of action.

Still, at some point on the road to self discovery, there's no turning back. It seems that the universe steps in and forces you to deal with all those things you are trying so hard not to face. For me, I slowly became attracted to books about Chronic Fatigue Syndrome, Fibromyalgia and pain management. Each title I read armed me with new information and some potential strategies.

In particular, I found strength and solace in three books. The first of these important resources was *Trigger Point Therapy for Myofascial Pain*. This is an extremely technical work meant for massage practitioners and pain management specialists. Even with the anatomy training that I gained as an archaeologist, I did not fully comprehend the information in this guide. Actually, I don't think I really even needed to grasp this depth of meaning at the time. What this title provided for me was full colour diagrams of those trigger points that the sports medicine specialist had tested on me so many years before. Now I could take my time and actually see where these spots were on my body.

I spent quite a bit of time finding each point and noticing that indeed the majority of these points were still tender, despite that my symptoms didn't seem as obvious as they had been when I first started this quest. As I worked through the illustrations, I also realized that my bouts of pain tended to start in these very specific areas and then traveled along the various muscle groups. Often, when the flare-ups were prolonged or the pain extremely bad, new trigger points in nearby muscle groups would be added into the mix.

What a revelation! I could actually see how my pain acted and how it spread. Instead of thinking of my pain as some sort of mysterious demon taking over my body, I began thinking of my symptoms as a button that gets stuck in the on position. If that mechanism failed to right itself, then eventually other body systems would be affected as well.

Now I just needed to figure out how to get my system to turn off at the right times. I tried massaging the trigger points as set out in this book, but frankly had very little success, even with the tennis ball massage treatment. Many of my most tender spots were and still are in my back and my neck where it is extremely difficult to reach with any sort of precision. Similarly, I didn't find the exercises provided all that useful either.

Still, that first book got me to pick up another one, *Fibromyalgia and Myofascial Pain: A Survival Manual*. This guide was written by an author who actually has Fibromyalgia and who was a wealth of knowledge without any trace of judgment (or pity). From the very first pages, I felt a kinship to the author. Yes, she had Fibromyalgia and yes sometimes life was hell for her, but she was looking for a way to live a happy, contented life despite her limitations. Moreover, unlike me, this person didn't hate the Fibromyalgia; it was merely just a fact of life, a challenge.

I learned many important things from this resource. As I read through all of the co-existing conditions and early symptoms that people don't tend to notice about Fibromyalgia, I realized that I was a pretty classic case of Fibromyalgia (if there is such as thing). I'd had plenty of allergies as a child. As a teen, I was diagnosed with Endometriosis and Renauld's Syndrome. I have always had bouts of insomnia, sleep apnea, calf cramps, and horrible headaches. At the depth of winter, every January for as long as I can remember, I've had an episode of deep depression.

These symptom lists made me really start to think. I began to realize that the sports medicine specialist had really known her stuff. I most definitely had Fibromyalgia. Not Multiple Sclerosis. Moreover, Fibromyalgia wasn't something that I got because I was stressed about my father-in-law's surgery, I dared to go back to school, or because I gained forty-five pounds in the process. Since I was six months old (my first medically recorded indication of allergies), I may have been showing a predisposition to Fibromyalgia. I might have even been destined to get Chronic Fatigue Syndrome and Fibromyalgia.

What a concept! My health issues started to take on a whole new light. I wasn't sick because of anything I did or didn't do. These conditions didn't sneak up on me to steal my happy life away just as things were beginning to get good. My health issues were merely medical conditions, just illness (read weakness) in the body.

Immediately, some of my anxieties started to dissipate. I started to let go of the worry of full disability and the potential of a wheelchair. At this point, I was almost a decade into my journey. Despite my deepest fears, my worst case scenarios, and that I rarely did anything to take care of my symptoms, I was living a fairly normal life. Yes, sometimes my pain got pretty bad, especially in my back, left hip, and head. Sometimes, I didn't sleep much, nothing new there. Dealing with fibrofog was extremely irritating. In spite of all this, I had managed to work, keep a house, and take care of myself without help. My conditions hadn't steadily gotten worse to a point where I was totally dependent upon my family. I wasn't as independent or as perfect as I would like to be but my life really wasn't all that bleak either.

One thing gnawed at me though. I still equated illness with weakness. I took to heart the many times that people told me that their back hurt too (from overexertion or a strain) or that they were tired (from drinking too much the night before or stress from work) but it didn't affect *their* work. They could still work full-time. I didn't look disabled? What was wrong with me? Strange but it wasn't so much the thought of having to work around challenges in my life that really got to me. It was the thought of being seen as weak, limited, inferior, flawed, or imperfect.

The next book I read, *Healing Pain*, gave me some amazing insight into pain. This resource looked at both the physical and emotional aspects of chronic pain. Until I read this work, I had no idea that chronic pain was any different from regular pain. The difference is so incredibly obvious that I had never even thought about it. Regular pain (acute) is associated with a specific event (a break, strain, illness, etc) so when the healing is complete, the problem goes away.

Chronic pain, on the other hand, is never really healed so if it goes away it's only a bit of a reprieve. You know that eventually the problem will be back with a vengeance. The body and the mind never truly get a rest and never really get a chance to recuperate before the next flare-up.

Needless to say, the body and the mind get drained, which naturally leads to a depressed state.

Wow! I wasn't just whiney and weak. Not only was my pain real, but the nature of these symptoms had distinct effects upon my body and my psyche. Again, I was normal (for chronic pain sufferers).

It seemed to me that all of the resources that I had been reading actually had a common theme. Whatever your health issues, you could find strategies to make your life liveable. The symptoms still might be there, but in regaining some aspect of control in your situation, you could regain independence, hope, and maybe even achieve a little happiness.

I realized that, with some help, I too might live a pretty decent life. With this goal in mind, I began searching for potential strategies. This journey would lead me to join a few discussion groups.

This simple act had an effect that I never could have imagined. Each time I read the discussion emails (and there were literally hundreds each day), I met people like myself: individuals in pain, suffering, confused, and really needing someone to understand that they weren't crazy or lazy. These people, like me, just wanted to be loved and live a good life, exactly like every other person in the world. They weren't flawed or despicable because these conditions had taken over their lives. They were just human beings trying their best to deal with what life had dealt them. I wasn't alone. There were thousands of others who understood exactly what I was going through because they had either gone through or were going through exactly the same things as me. I was normal!

8 The Big Symptoms

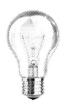

"You gain strength, courage and confidence by every experience in which you really stop to look fear in the face. You are able to say to yourself, 'I lived through this horror. I can take the next thing that comes along' ...you must do the thing you think you cannot do."
—Eleanor Roosevelt (1884-1962)

As I continued to read through and participate in the group discussions, I came to realize that I had already made some pretty big strides in taking charge of my health. Although I still suffered with small problems on most days and had slightly larger, more debilitating symptoms on occasion, it had been a long time since I had suffered from a major flare-up that lasted weeks at a time or that caused mobility issues.

During much of my suffering thus far, I hadn't been consciously coming up with strategies to cope with my health. Mostly, I ignored any problems until they threatened to become visible to others. Then, basically out of fear that others might see my imperfections, I would do something drastic to get my body back out of the danger zone.

Yet, in the process, I had come up with a good deal of emergency strategies. In fact, I had actually already collected a whole array of ready-made solutions and coping mechanisms for different circumstances. When my legs collapsed, when I had debilitating fatigue, my bowels shut down, or when I experienced overwhelming fibrofog, I had not only figured out ways to cope with the situation at hand but had also learned a few quick tricks that could get my body back on the mend.

I admit that in the beginning of my exploration, my means were rather crude and not very kind or loving. I tended to self medicate with vitamins, herbs, over the counter drugs, and food. Although I did do a little research on everything I was taking and did put some thought into drug interactions, I was quite willing to experiment on myself like a guinea pig in hopes that something would eventually work. I was eager to take advice from anyone who had written an article, had a webpage, or thought they might have some sort of idea. Looking back, I realize that my actions were utterly ridiculous, irresponsible, and horribly dangerous.

I think for the most part, my hypothesis at the time was that if I shocked my body to a point where it either gave up completely or began getting better, that an instinctual survival mechanism would kick in and I would get better. Possibly, I also felt that I couldn't feel any worse so I was willing to try anything.

Fortunately, my methodologies eventually became more kind, loving, and caring. For each crisis symptom, I created what evolved into three distinct parts that combine to form a whole healing strategy. The first layer of these methodologies is generally a coping mechanism that allows me to deal with the actual situation at hand. For instance, when my legs collapse, I rely upon my cane George to support me so that I can stay somewhat mobile. For bouts of debilitating fatigue, I take naps to reduce the effects of sleep deprivation. When my bowels shut down, I use a warm magic bag to reduce the localized pain and discomfort until my system gets back to normal. As for fibrofog, my coping mechanism is a good editor who critiques all of my writing to see if I actually said what I meant to say.

The second part of my process is always some form of meditation. When I have a flare-up, I tend to get quite anxious. I immediately begin remembering the time that this symptom led to a particularly bad bout and wonder if this incident is going to lead to a similar end. Alternatively, I worry that this incident could foreshadow loss of mobility, reduced independence, and complete disability. This might be the thing that pushes me into that wheelchair, permanently. I believe that often just sitting in these negative thoughts adds even more stress to my body and mind. In turn, this extra stress may actually assure that these horrible fantasies do happen.

Meditation seems to calm me down and keeps me more positive. The process centers me and makes me realize that "this too will pass." Furthermore, I find that while meditating, my body and my mind relaxes. Fibromyalgia tends to create tenderness in my muscles. I notice that when I become tense or upset about this feeling, my muscles tighten up even more, creating greater pain. However, when I meditate, my muscles loosen up, reducing the likelihood of increased suffering caused by tense-ness. Likewise, my anxiety about my lack of a restful sleep tends to create a cycle of greater likelihood of insomnia and fatigue. Meditation, however, distracts me from my anxiety. I can then relax enough to fall into a restful sleep.

My meditation sessions tend to follow two main lines of thinking: focus on the present moment, and positive visualizations for the future. Al-though the actual steps and procedures can vary substantially, sessions that focus on the present moment tend to draw my attention inward. For instance, when I concentrate on each breath from that initial drawing as it flows down to my abdomen and then back out, all of my other worries and thoughts naturally dissipate. Basically, I give no attention to all those nasty thoughts and worries so they simply fall away. Really, it doesn't matter what I focus on, it could be a candle, waves, a pretty picture, a sound, a single thought, an affirmation, or a mantra. Anything that keeps my attention for a period of time seems to work.

I also find that my focus need not even be on one particular thing. I regularly do several relaxation mediations where I focus on certain parts of my body in turn. In one such exercise, I contract and relax specific groups of muscles, one set at a time: my feet, my calves, my thighs, etc. In another variation, I imagine warmth and relaxation gradually expand-ing from my feet to my head like a warm loving blanket being pulled over my body.

Visualization tends to be more purposeful. I use visualizations to en-courage a specific positive outcome. For instance, I may imagine my pain being squeezed from, pulled out of, or dissipated from my body. Alterna-tively, I may concentrate on how my body feels when I have a lot of energy. Thus, I draw my attention to the good things that I want to hap-pen rather then thinking about all of the bad things that could occur or have taken place in the past. In doing so, I focus on manifesting positive outcomes rather then reinforcing negative thinking cycles.

Over time, I have created a variety of different mediations and visuali-zations for relaxation, pain management, and manifesting positive outcomes. For most of these exercises, I have created several variations so that I can easily practice meditation or visualization no matter what my physical and mental abilities are at the time. Given my wide range of potential health issues on any given day, this flexibility is crucial.

At the beginning of my journey through Chronic Fatigue Syndrome and Fibromyalgia, I tended to focus entirely on meditation to release negative thoughts, refocus myself, and gain a positive perspective. Once I started to come out of my deepest depths of denial, I also started journaling. I now take time every day to journal, but I make a special effort to write when I am in the midst of a bad bout. In both situations, I record my feelings, my worries, my hopes, and my dreams. I find that this action helps me release my anxieties in a safe way (as opposed to yelling at my husband or being rude to the clerk at the supermarket). Basically, once I have written down my thoughts, I have given myself permission to feel the depth of these situations, learn from them, and then to let go.

The process of writing often reminds me that most of my horror scenarios come from a place of fear. I am afraid that the pain in my legs will spread and get worse. I am worried that I won't be able to walk someday. I am terrified that eventually I might not be able to work or be self-sufficient.

Yes, these things might happen, but they haven't occurred yet. Until they do, if they ever do, I will try to live my life to the fullest. I can't very well change the things that took place in the past. As for the future, I will have to deal with any potential situation then. I can't possibly prepare myself for every horrible scenario that might come up in my life, so there is always the possibility that I will be surprised by a situation and have to fumble to come to grips with it. The best I can do is realize that I've already dealt with a lot of difficult challenges in my life and faced them. The result wasn't always pretty but I'm still alive and breathing.

I find that with these terror stories out of my way, I can see what really matters to me. I can see the good in my life and the sorts of activities that I can do right now. I can see the things in my life that I do because I think I'm supposed to do them, and I can then make a conscious decision to place my energy and efforts in places that are more meaningful to me. Some days I only have enough energy to do one or two things. My "to do" list might include a lot of things like cleaning, laundry, making meals or the like, but my energy is valuable. I see more merit in writing another chapter of this book, spending time with my kids, or going for a nice walk. So what if the house is a mess, it'll just get that way again anyway.

Another supportive strategy that I have recently begun using is Reiki. Reiki is a bioelectrical methodology to aid stress relief, pain management, and to improve relaxation. Reiki was originally based upon ancient Buddhist healing practices where life energy is used to heal physical, mental, emotional, and spiritual pain while filtering out negativity and creating greater balance in the body systems. This process can be achieved either through hands-on massage or through distance healings whereby the energies are sent through the various aura layers or the magnetism of the combined atoms that make up the human body.

There are many variations of Reiki that tend to combine traditional healing techniques of various cultures and the original form of Reiki. Thus, those with a Christian background may be attracted to Reiki that has been intermeshed with the healing power of Angels or the power of the Christ Consciousness, while those who resonate with more New Age beliefs may find Reiki combined with aura therapy or chakra balancing more to their liking. By the same token, those with a scientific background may be more comfortable discussing alpha waves or magnetic fields in relation to Reiki energies.

In my mind, Reiki does two important things. First, whether I self heal or have a friend send Reiki energies, the process makes me stop and take active control of my health. For the entire time it takes to do a session (thirty minutes to an hour), I sit and allow myself to be completely relaxed. I think of nothing except my body feeling healthier. Thus, like meditation, during Reiki sessions I am allowing myself a bit of a break from all those nasty worries and dread fantasy potentials that I tend to put myself through.

Furthermore, most Reiki practitioners will tell you that the source of Reiki energies is unconditional love. Depending upon their own personal beliefs, these individuals may call that source God, the inner self, the universe, I Am, or a thousand other things but it all comes down to unconditional love. The power to heal is through love. The thought of that concept is extremely powerful and thought provoking to me. I see the energies that move through me as evidence that I am loveable. Even when my head aches, even during the worst bout of fibrofog, I am still worthy of love and I am a valuable human being. Really, what more could I ask?

During the worst of my crisis symptoms, sometimes I still need a little extra help. It is at this point that I turn to the third layer of my emergency strategy plan. This aspect of my process is always something external: a prescribed drug, an over the counter medicine, a vitamin, an herbal supplement, or other external form of medication.

Although I am not completely adverse to prescribed medications, I still shy away from them. This is merely a personal preference and not any sort of value judgment on modern medicine or medical practices. I simply don't find a good deal of comfort in these approaches. I don't like taking a bunch of pills each day, feeling dependent upon them or the doctor to prescribe them. It makes me feel like someone else has control of my destiny—that someone else holds the power to give me a happy, healthy life or take it away if they so deem. I may still be in a bit of denial but I prefer thinking and feeling that, come what may, I can determine what my life should look and feel like. I may not be in complete control of my symptoms, but I can choose to be content and to live my life to the fullest.

To this end, my external medications tend to be over-the-counter drugs, food, vitamins, or herbal supplements. For instance, I have noticed that one of the chief causes of my leg pain and weakness is actually swelling of the knee joints. Therefore, when this situation arises, I use Arthritic Rub A535 on my knees. This rub lotion seems to reduce that swelling often enough so that my joints can move again.

For debilitating fatigue, I still rely upon Bee Pollen, which gradually gets my energy back to a more normal level. For quick pick me ups, I make myself a concoction of hot water, blackstrap molasses and lemon juice. This drink lifts the fatigue quite quickly but doesn't seem to bring me down as fast as a chocolate bar or something else sweet.

The energy enhancing effect of my molasses-lemon drink is actually a side benefit. I found this concoction while looking for a strategy to deal with my bowels shutting down. I had tried everything from laxatives and fiber to prunes and colon cleanses but nothing seemed to work. With the laxatives and food supplements, I just got bloated and my intestine pain intensified without any sort of relief. I think this happened mostly because I wasn't constipated. My bowels had simply shut down. Nothing much happened with the colon cleanses. My system still stayed as it was for a few more days until it decided to return to normal.

The only thing that worked (periodically) was chocolate milkshakes. I really like this cure because I really enjoy chocolate milk shakes, but the truth is that probably the only reason this solution did work was that the milkshakes contained milk and I am lactose intolerant. Basically, by drinking the milkshake, I was sending irritants into my system and expecting it to fall apart or fight. Despite that it tasted good, this was definitely not a very loving plan.

Today, I use the molasses-lemon drink, which is far gentler and doesn't cause all the intestinal pain. I also find that the herbal supplements poria and magnolia or regularly eating probiotic yogurt also do the same thing, but they work better over the long term rather than as a quick fix. In the midst of a bout, I am not ready to wait three or four extra days to feel relief. By the by, I still drink milkshakes sometimes, but I take some of those lactase enzyme pills to reduce the intestinal pain, bloating and diarrhea.

I am still looking for a good medicine for fibrofog. Over the long term, Ginkgo Biloba does helps somewhat, but is not a particularly good quick fix. This herbal supplement improves memory and focus. However, it does not help with the dyslexic aspects of Fibromyalgia (confusing opposites, mixing up numbers, and differentiating directions). Plus, I sometimes find it hard to remember to take pills regularly when I'm in the midst of a bad bout.

9 Individual Strategies

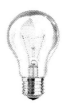

"They say that time changes things, but you actually have to change them yourself."
—Andy Warhol (1928-1987)

So began a timid line of research unlike any other I had done to that point. Instead of frantically focusing on some sort of achievement in order to hide from my pain and despair, I was willing to walk straight into that chaos. I was prepared (tentatively at first perhaps) to face my health issues, my fears, and myself, come what may.

I knew that the risks would definitely be worth it if I could only find myself in a better place. Besides, I had come to the point in my investigations where I couldn't really turn back. I couldn't live in denial forever, continually beating myself up every day for not being perfect. My psyche, my self esteem, and maybe even my sanity couldn't take much more. The damage and abuse that I had piled upon myself had already threatened to destroy me forever. The strong, independent, driven woman I had been had slowly turned into a tiny shadow scared of living.

So, although I had no idea what I'd find at the end of my journey, I proceeded. I was willing to try in hopes of finding peace and contentment. Deep down inside, I also prayed that I would find myself and that person would be someone I could love, value and respect.

I realized that I already had a good foundation of ready-made strategies to cope with, control, and reduce the worst of my flare-ups. Now I just needed to expand this knowledge. Several of the books that I had read (most notably *Fibromyalgia and Myofascial Pain: A Survival Manual*, and *Healing Pain*) had suggested that the best way to deal with chronic illness and pain was through keeping records of symptoms and then experimenting with strategies to cope with these health issues. This plan seemed like a good way to start so I decided to keep a daily record of my health issues. My intention was that I would keep a journal about what I was feeling and where my pain, fatigue or other ills were centered. In addition to this information, I also noted the intensity, things that I felt might have brought on the bout, anything that seemed to make the episode worse, and strategies that I tried to alleviate the problem.

So I began. At first, my investigations were rather simplistic and somewhat naïve. I fantasized that my studies would create a great list of symptoms and treatments. Once completed, whenever I suffered from one of these conditions, I would simply look through the file, find the appropriate solution, and feel better instantly.

Don't get me wrong, I still believe that the intent behind my exploration is valid, and I adamantly continue my process of compiling strategies. Experimenting and trying to find ways of coping with symptoms is definitely a worthwhile task. How else will I find out what exactly is going to relieve my ills? Waiting for the magic pain relief fairy or hoping that an all encompassing cure will fall in my lap simply isn't very realistic. I truly believe that taking control and responsibility of my health issues is the only way that I can rediscover my independence and take back my life.

Nonetheless, this line of experimentation is not simple and is an ongoing (perhaps never ending) undertaking. There are often many ways of dealing with a single symptom. This makes the process extremely complicated, but there is some good news in this complexity. Having choice means that I can pick a single strategy or combination of tactics that also suits my emotional and psychological needs. Ultimately, I can tailor my health plan to suit me.

For instance, I sometimes suffer from bouts of depression related to my conditions. As I mentioned in a previous chapter, my doctor thought that the only solution to this problem was drug therapy. This treatment, although it may work, is something that I was and still am personally uncomfortable with. In fact, if given the choice, I tend to stay away from drugs, pills, or even vitamins of any kind. This doesn't mean that I don't think that these strategies wouldn't work on me, that I would never choose these alternatives if they would benefit me, or that I think that others shouldn't try these solutions. On the contrary, I think that we all have to find means that work for us and that suit our very individualized situations. Our circumstances, symptoms, needs, and personalities are unique so why wouldn't our treatment options be just as varied?

To add to the intricacy of my symptom strategy research, I noted several very interesting potentially useful clues. There were patterns, lots of patterns. The great thing about recording daily changes was that I could see in black and white that sometimes a small, seemingly unimportant symptom (such as a pulling feeling in my right ear, a slight ache at the base of my back, or pain in my left hip) could quite easily turn into a full blown flareup that would spread to other areas of my body and mind.

This discovery led, and continues to lead, to other lines of experimentation. For instance, I try to watch out for those little twinges that tend to turn into full blown bouts of fatigue, pain, or fibrofog. When I recognize these signs, I look for ways to deal them before they turn into bigger issues. This may sound a little bit like chasing a ghost in the dark but there is actually some intelligent thought in this process.

It would seem that that little ear pull is like the engine of a train. That engine can be followed by any number of cars. The same is true of my seemingly little health issues. Small signs are often followed by other symptoms. That ear pull might lead to headaches and pain in the extremities. Worst case scenario, this could lead to my legs giving way and pain lasting for weeks, which causes me to fly right into a bad flare-up of fatigue and insomnia. Then, I'm back to dealing with full blown Chronic Fatigue Syndrome and Fibromyalgia.

But not all engines have to carry a full load of cars and not all small symptoms have to lead to long bouts of disability. I often find that by taking care of that little problem, I don't have to deal with a larger bout that could have potentially caused disability. Thus, if I simply stop, relax, meditate, and place a nice warm magic bag on my ear, then the ear pull feeling disappears and that's the end of my problem. Going back to my train analogy, I tell the engineer that no cars are needed and he simply goes on his merry way.

Actually being able to reduce the intensity and duration of my health conditions is a huge boon. Yes, I have to be more aware of those little things and be willing to take care of them right away, but it does relieve the possibility of long periods of debilitating pain and fatigue. Although somewhat limiting, this process does give me an ounce of freedom and ultimately reduces the feeling that disability is inevitable.

I also feel like I have some aspect of control and independence back in my life. This is perhaps the most important benefit of this exercise. My health problems often rob me of control over my destiny. Often, my life seemed dependent upon my husband, my family, and the medical profession for my care. They made all the decisions and I had no choice in the matter. Sometimes it seemed like all my hopes and dreams were in the hands of the disease. It could determine whether I lived a happy life or whether I diminished until there would be nothing left but a bitter old woman.

Now, by using my plan, I have some say. I have a little control back in my life. I may have to deal with those small symptoms on their terms and my strategies don't work every time, but I am back taking responsibility for myself and my own care. I decide what methods suit me best. I determine what works and what doesn't. It's my life, my responsibility, my care, and my choice. Now, that's freedom, and a life potentially worth living.

In my investigations, I have noticed that of all the health issues that I experience in my day to day life, there are a few that seem to be the most prevalent. These symptoms are fatigue, depression, joint swelling, leg pain, back pain, foot pain, chest pain, headaches, fibrofog, and weight gain. Over time, I have kept records of my experiences with each of these problems and I have gained quite a lot of insight into them.

It would seem that each of these types of flare-ups have a fairly predictable pattern of progression. For instance, my bouts of fatigue usually start off innocently enough with a single night of unrecuperative sleep. I find that if I am not careful to have a nap the next day to make up for the lost sleep, or if I go to bed a little tense the next night, I will quickly find myself falling into a cycle of debilitating insomnia.

The same is true of my pain symptoms. The majority of these symptoms start in one spot (my hips, my feet, the frame of my back, etc). If I ignore these small warnings, then the feeling expands out to other related areas: hip pain moves down the legs, foot pain moves up the leg, back pain leads to chest pain, etc. Moreover, as they spread, the intensity worsens. Thus, what starts out as a pain rating of 3 out of 10 (mildly irritating) quickly becomes 5 out of ten (somewhat debilitating) and then grows to 8 out of 10 (disabling).

If left unchecked, one symptom can lead to or exasperate another set of symptoms. The best examples in my experience are weight gain and depression. When I am in severe pain or am feeling insecure about my independence as is common with Chronic Fatigue Syndrome and Fibromyalgia, I just want to feel better. At the time, I really don't care how I feel better, I just want it now. I can easily see how someone in a similar situation might turn to drugs or alcohol to ease the suffering. I find solace in food. Most of the time, I don't even realize what I am doing. In the midst of a bout, at a certain point (usually when the symptoms get to be 5 out of 10 or more), I start to crave chocolate and carbohydrates. As the pain increases, so do the cravings. Moreover, when in the midst of these intense experiences, I never quite feel full so I am constantly hungry. Add to this that regular exercise is extremely difficult when my symptoms are debilitating, it is no wonder that I start to gain a little extra weight.

My depression symptoms follow a similar vein. Once my pain or fatigue issues become unbearable, I get anxious over my lack of independence. I start to worry that this might be the time that my symptoms don't go away. Perhaps, this will be the beginning of the end for me. I won't be able to lose those ten extra pounds (okay, more honestly, twenty pounds), I won't be able to work, and I won't be able to care for myself. I see visions of my husband having to drag me out of the bathtub because I can't do it myself. He'd start to see me as a burden and wouldn't want to be with me anymore. My children would then have to take on the burden. No-one wants their children to give up their dreams to care for them. As this detrimental line of thinking continues, I get deeper and deeper into that dark place where I wonder if life is even worth living.

Given the terrible potential of these recognizable cycles, I have worked hard to come up with ways to deal with them. I believe that probably the most important thing in these situations is to notice my issues as early as possible, preferably before the symptoms get to 5 out of 10. To me, it makes perfectly logical sense that the earlier that I start working on alleviating a health issue, the less pain and suffering I have to endure.

Although I may not necessarily be able to completely get rid of any particular symptom, I find that I can often keep the entire flare-up at a level below 5 out of 10. Thus, for the most part, I can go about my regular daily routine without much disruption. For the most part, I can even convince myself that life with Chronic Fatigue Syndrome and Fibromyalgia is not that bad. Even though the symptoms aren't completely gone, I can pretty much continue to live my normal life. Ultimately, I have a more positive outlook on my life and my future.

As with my strategies in the previous chapter on crisis or emergency health concerns, I follow the same basic format in my explorations for individual symptoms. Again, I have a list of coping mechanisms, meditations and medications. Thus, when my hips starts to ache a little, I recognize that I need to rest my legs and either place a warm magic bag on the area or use some Rub A535 Formula on it. Then, I make time for a little meditation, journaling, and some Reiki.

I find that a quick reaction is especially important with my chest pains. The first couple of times I had these symptoms, I thought I was having a heart attack. I was absolutely terrified. I went to the doctor and she really didn't give me any substantial answers. I came away unsure if I had indeed had a heart attack or not. As I mentioned earlier in this book, I later learned from a discussion group posting that these pains were nothing to be concerned with, that they were just another fact of living with Chronic Fatigue Syndrome and Fibromyalgia. Since that point, my mother and oldest daughter have both mentioned that they get these squeezing chest feelings. My daughter's doctor gently assured her that she was not having a heart attack and that basically the neurons in the brain become overloaded and fire randomly until the body resets itself naturally.

Despite that I now know that my chest pains are not at all dangerous, if the episode lasts for any amount of time, I start to panic. Therefore, as soon as I feel that ache in the frame of my back, I heat up my magic bag, make myself a nice warm cup of chamomile tea, and find someone to talk to so my mind stays busy. Alternatively, if I am alone when the incident occurs, I begin to meditate. These actions seem to reduce both the duration and intensity of the bout.

A few of these individual symptoms such as fatigue, fibrofog and joint swelling relate directly to emergency situations that I discussed in the previous sections. The only difference in my investigations at the individual symptom level is that I now look to stop the progression of problems before it reaches that crisis level. Thus, instead of waiting for the joint swelling to reduce my mobility to the point where I can't walk, I immediately rest and elevate my legs, rub Arthritic Rub A535 Formula on my swollen knee joints, and begin my mediations and Reiki sessions. This way, my health issues need never get to that emergency point.

10 My Own Worst Enemy

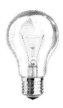

> "The hardest thing to learn in life is which bridge to cross and which to burn."
>
> —David Russell (1953-)

This line of exploration and research has been the catalyst for a whole new way of thinking for me. I no longer feel that Chronic Fatigue Syndrome and Fibromyalgia are ruling my life. Now, there is hope. I have some sense of control over the direction my life takes. I may not stop every small symptom before it turns into a larger flare-up, but I know that I have some direct effect on my health. Furthermore, I find that even when I do suffer from symptoms and bad bouts, I tend to focus more on what strategies I could try to reduce the problem. This leaves me less time to beat myself up over feeling like I'm flawed or weak because I have these health issues. Those lines of thoughts just seemed to make the situation seem all the more bleak anyway.

My investigations have also led to another important area of discovery. As I endeavoured to find the earliest small symptom, I started to notice certain events or particular circumstances that tended to predate even these little issues. Stress, lack of sleep, overexertion, an unbalanced routine, other illness, menstruation, and weather changes were the most common symptom catalysts.

Immediately from this listing, it may seem obvious that the majority of my flare-ups are actually somewhat preventable. If I simply listened to my body, I would realize that I was pushing my mind and body too far. I would say that enough is enough. I would take a break when I needed it. I would take a short nap. I would say no to unrealistic deadlines. I would take on only what I could realistically accomplish in the time given. In short, I would be more kind and loving to myself.

This concept may seem obvious to many people, but frankly I just didn't see the signs. Sometimes, I still don't. Yes, I knew that working twenty hours straight with no sleep trying to get three projects done before an unrealistic deadline probably wasn't the healthiest way to live. Still, I had myself convinced that in order to be successful I had to put in more time and effort than everyone else. Again, I saw and Fibromyalgia as evidence that I was a flawed being. I was essentially a born loser and sooner or later everyone else would find that out if I wasn't careful.

Thus, I spent every waking second trying to prove that I was valuable and invulnerable. I had so much to overcome. I needed to prove myself. Any way that I seemed to look at the situation, I felt I had to "suck it up" and work harder to validate myself. What an absolute crock!

I now know that I was setting myself up for failure. The more I stressed or tired myself trying to do more in a shorter time, the more I was increasing my risk of having a bout that would impede my progress. Yes, I did manage to get a lot done in some very short periods of time, but I likely would have gotten the same amount accomplished if I'd just paced myself better. Perhaps, I would have found that I was even more productive when I took breaks, dealt with my stress, or generally listened when my body said it was nearing its limit. I do find that after taking some time away from my work I am far more energetic, creative, and even the most difficult task seems just a bit easier.

Of course, changing the entire way I think, behave, and react to my body's natural signs is a work in progress. As I write this paragraph, I am dog sick with the flu. At times, I am coughing so hard that I can hardly catch my breath and my chest hurts from all the hacking. I should be in bed sleeping. I know it. It's extremely obvious that I should probably wait until I am better to start writing again. The writing will still be there tomorrow or next week.

That would be a logical thing to do, but my mind doesn't always work that way. I know that I am nearing the end of my Chronic Fatigue Syndrome and Fibromyalgia story to this point and will soon finish writing the text of this book. My natural reaction is that the moment I see an achievement nearing its end, I get focused and fixated on finishing it. I am like a dog with his favourite bone. Right now, I can't seem to think about anything except getting this writing completed. I can't sleep. I can't rest. I just find myself drawn to typing away endlessly.

I find myself making up arbitrary (unrealistic) deadlines for myself. Maybe I can get done writing before the end of the week. Then, I could take x number of days to edit. Then, the publication process (submission, waiting for a reply, editing, etc) could be done by such and such a day. Then, the actual book might be released by such and such a date.

The worst part is that I see myself doing these unhealthy things and know I need to stop. I know that I am setting myself up for a really bad flare-up. I realize that ultimately finishing this book, editing, and the submission process will be as long or short as it takes. I can't hurry that. Nor would I want to, not really. I would hate to have put all this time and effort into my story only to have it rushed and incomplete at the end. That would cheapen and invalidate my experiences. I may as well have not even started to type in the first place, if I were going to sabotage my work in that way.

Again, perhaps this is the reason that I have Chronic Fatigue Syndrome and Fibromyalgia. I haven't yet learned to listen to my body when it says enough is enough. I just can't seem to police myself. Maybe, it's time to make a smart start. It's time to make better choices. It's time to put my health first all of the time, not just when it's convenient. I think I'm going to make myself a nice cup of Sleepy Time Tea and then have a nap.

11 Prevention is the Best Policy

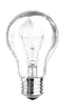

"What is necessary to change a person is to change his awareness of himself."

—Abraham H. Maslow (1908-1970)

Ultimately, I think that learning to listen to my body and making a constant effort to put my health ahead of everything else in my life is going to be the best overall strategy to deal with Chronic Fatigue Syndrome and Fibromyalgia. I may not be able to stop myself from menstruating and potentially have a bad flare-up. I may not be able to control the rapid weather changes that come with the Chinooks that occur in Calgary. Still, like the individual symptoms that I have investigated so far, I have found that I can reduce the likelihood of bad bouts and limit the debilitating effects of my health issues.

It has taken me some time to come up with just the right mixture of prevention strategies. Like everything that I do, I tend to start off with extremely unrealistic expectations and then try to force myself to conform to these ideals. For instance, my first exercise programs were heinous. For some reason, I felt that I needed to exercise every day for at least a half hour and then take a long walk each day as well. The first couple of days on this program, I actually managed to accomplish these tasks. I hurt all over and I was tired, but I still pushed. Inevitably though, I caused myself to have a bad flare-up so that I couldn't exercise for a few weeks. After this, I had to start from scratch once again.

After more times that I'd like to admit to, I finally realized that this action was a cycle of self abuse. I had to come up with a more realistic plan. My exercise schedule is now far more flexible. I really enjoy being outside in the fresh air, so when the weather is good I try to take regular walks on the pathways near my house.

During the winter and on cold or rainy days, I make use of my Gazelle Edge Glider (www.FitnessQuest.com). I find it is easier on my knees and joints than most other pieces of exercise equipment, while still providing a good workout. My goal is generally fifteen to twenty minutes of exercise per day. However, if I'm having a challenging body day or my schedule is going to be really hectic, I usually break my session up into ten minute shifts between other jobs. This way I still get the stress relief and energy from having a workout without hurting myself.

I find that exercise and fresh air help my overall outlook on my life. I guess being somewhat active, even during the worst of my symptoms, reminds me that Chronic Fatigue Syndrome and Fibromyalgia can't take everything from me. I can still be vital, adventurous, and even a bit of fun.

In addition to exercise and fresh air, a healthy body needs a nutritious diet. Like most people, I have tried a number of different diet regimes and finding the right one for me hasn't been easy. I had some success with a gluten-free diet. I found that the food I ate while on this plan did indeed make me feel better and I didn't suffer from intestinal cramping. I also managed to release 15 pounds in a fairly short length of time.

However, there were a few flaws in this system that I just couldn't mesh with my lifestyle. My family does not share my adventurous nature when it comes to food. It's hard enough to get them to eat a stir fry, and they completely refuse to even try tofu. For family meals, gluten-free fare is definitely out. During the entire time I worked through my plan, I was making multiple meals. With my energy being a valuable resource, I found this quite difficult and disruptive.

The other major problem with gluten-free cooking was that there were very few ready to cook choices at my local supermarket. If you look carefully at the labels, you will see that almost everything has some sort of wheat additive including tofu, ketchup, Soya sauce, chocolate bars, etc. Those foods that were gluten-free were twice or three times the price of the regular version. My budget is pretty tight so this really put me off. Thus, I spent much of my time on the plan eating fresh vegetables and fruit. This is not a bad start in and of itself.

From there, I started to cut out carbohydrates completely. It was a fairly short stint because this plan was completely unsuitable for me. I am not a big meat eater. I eat chicken and maybe a little pork or fish every so often but for the most part I could live without meat. I do like tofu and find that the meatless meatballs, burgers, chicken, pepperoni, etc that they sell at the supermarket taste pretty good. I get a variety of tastes but my body doesn't feel sick or bloated afterward.

The second part of a carbohydrate-free diet that I found difficult was the lack of carbohydrates. The nature of carbohydrates is that they increase your serotonin levels. Serotonin is the hormone in your body that makes you feel good, your happy hormone if you will. That's why carbohydrates tend to make excellent comfort food. When I go through my worst bouts (where I can't see the end in sight) I tend to turn to food for comfort, specifically those high in complex carbohydrates.

When I first started this particular plan, I thought that my cravings of carbohydrates were my body's way of rebelling. I stayed firm, trying to force myself to adhere to my regime. I subsequently became depressed and extremely hungry. I was in very serious danger of going into full blown binge mode and wrecking all my hard work.

Fortunately, I came to realize that a carbohydrate-free life was not for me. My nutritional plan, like every other strategy that I have come up with, has to be tailored to my needs and my lifestyle. It needs to fit me.

This fact really hit home with me when I read a book called *The Four Day Win*. This wasn't a diet book per se. It did not present a single exercise or health regime. Instead, this guide dealt with the underlying psychology of the weight loss-gain yoyo that we all experience.

Simply put, I realized I was trying to fit myself into someone else's version of ideal. When I chose a diet, my focus was on losing weight rather than eating to feel healthy. I moved more and ate less but I never actually stopped to listen to my body. Often, in the process, I hurt myself by trying to exercise for x number of minutes when my muscles weren't used to doing any exercise at all. In the end, I just hurt all over and felt starved. Not surprisingly, the plan ultimately failed.

My current health care plan is fairly simple. I am trying to learn to listen when my body is hungry and then I feed it. Then, the really tough part, I only eat until I am no longer hungry. My body seems to know what it really needs to be healthy and energetic. I find it will crave salad when I haven't been eating enough vegetables, or protein when I'm in need of a little extra strength and energy.

I find that this methodology works. I don't feel starved. Most importantly, I realized that a good deal of the food I consumed in the past was a complete waste. I wasn't hungry at all. I was stressed and overwhelmed. My body was craving comfort and a safe place. I normally found that comfort in food. No wonder my system got so mad when I tried to limit my food quantities and take away its carbohydrates. I had basically taken away its only coping mechanism and told it that I wasn't willing to listen to its problems. How absolutely horrible!

Once I realized what I had been doing to myself, I saw that my weight gain was not at all about my lack of exercise or the quantity of food I was consuming. The issue went much deeper. Funny, my issues seemed to be taking me back again and again to the exact same conclusion. I needed to be kind to myself and listen to my body. I had to stop all the self-loathing and self-judgement about what I perceived as flaws and start recognizing that I was just fine exactly as I was. I don't have to be someone else's version of perfect, busy, beautiful, smart, etc. I just have to fine within myself.

I now have a whole list of self-soothing activities that I practice on a regular basis. At least once a day, I journal and meditate. I tend to journal in the morning to get my focus straight for the day. It gives me the opportunity to stop and realize what my body has to say about my ability levels for the day. My first priority can then be to determine what strategies I need to use for my pain and fatigue symptoms on that particular day. My general goal is to keep the pain and fatigue below 5 out of 10 so that they are not debilitating or disruptive.

Journaling also helps me gauge how much work I can potentially get done in a single day. My energy levels vary quite significantly. I look at how much energy I have and how my body is feeling, and then I determine what I can get done in that particular day. I'm getting fairly good at estimating my limitations on regular and more difficult days. However, I still tend to overestimate for days that I feel very energetic. I still take on too much and not get the work complete or I finish the work and drain myself to the point that I have bad body days for the next few days. Balance is the key.

As noted, most of my health issue strategies also include some sort of journaling. I find that most of my symptoms bring up feelings of inadequacy, anger or blame. Although I do see Chronic Fatigue Syndrome and Fibromyalgia as boons, I still worry that it labels me as weak and may limit the potential success of my dreams. I like making use of journaling because it allows me to release some of my emotions and concerns in a safe way. Usually, in these cases, my entries start off with a lot of venting and raw emotion. Then, gradually I come back to myself and realize that the foundation of my feeling is almost always fear that something might happen that I can't handle. It is at this point that I remind myself of how truly adaptable I am. I know that I can get through almost anything that life throws at me. My actions or reactions may not be pretty or perfect but I will survive. Hell, I may even thrive a bit every now and then.

To help keep me centered, I try to take some time to meditate every day. Early on during my meditation practice, I realized the many benefits of these sessions. It was obvious even to me that I could go into the exercise feeling overwhelmed, stressed out, and hating the world but after I was done I always felt more positive and patient. Right away, I knew that this practice could be a great gift in my life.

Still, it has taken me many years to find a practical way to fit meditation into my daily life. I believe that the delay to integrate this practice was rather illustrative of the way that I used to think and act. I believe that I was extremely dogmatic. Everything in my life was black and white. There was no room for any gray. Either I fit into the ideal of perfect or I was a worthless human being. There was absolutely no room for being human, making mistakes, or growing. I had to be everything at all times.

At first, I took this outlook with me into my meditation. I had a Buddhist text that described how to undertake the process. I followed these words as if they were some sort of sacred law. The book said I should find a room just for meditation. I cleaned out my closet and sat on the floor. During the actual process, I was constantly aware of my body position, making sure I had the perfect straight back, that my lotus position was open enough, and that my tongue was in the right place. I was extremely militant when my mind wandered and constantly kept that in check. I also felt that the amount of meditation that I did each day somehow defined how well I was doing. Half an hour wasn't enough, one hour was better, but somewhere in my chaotic mind I felt that I should be practicing all day like some sort of fanatical monk.

How unrealistic can you get? Who has that kind of time? Who can even do a lotus position when their body pain is 7 out if 10? Thus, because of my perfectionism, my sessions become yet another way of punishing myself and proving that I was indeed a loser.

I'm so very glad that I didn't completely block mediation out of my life. Today it is my solace. It is my time to remind myself that all of the chaos, pain, and stress does not touch who I really am inside. The part that is me, that unchangeable part that some might call a soul, a life consciousness, or part of the one, is joyful in itself. Essentially, it is perfect. This aspect of me sees all the things that I experience as an interesting exploration. Look how this Tami body and mind react when x, y, z happens. Isn't that interesting? No judgments. No excuses. Just the pure joy of the experience.

What changed my mind, figuratively and literally? I'm really not completely sure if there was one thing that made the difference. The transition took a great deal of time. After I started meditation, I began doing a lot of research on different cultures. Simultaneously, I was working on my bachelor's degree in Archaeology. Thus, I was already spending a good deal of time learning about the lifeways of others.

I have always been intrigued with the lives of other people. I'm one of those beings who enjoys watching the biography channel and reads autobiographies of people that no one's every even heard about. Likely, given my nature, I was looking at ways to become like those I envied or trying to measure myself against those who were successful.

Studying other cultures was slightly different. One of my first university lectures taught about the danger of the western ethnocentric nature, basically believing that our culture holds the ultimate truth and all other beliefs or ways of doing things are beneath us. That in limiting our vision in this way we miss out the greater truth of these experiences. Essentially, we then cheapen the lives of individuals who depended upon us as archaeologists to tell their story.

I really took that message to heart. I took in information like a sponge. Each artefact, custom and belief became absolutely amazing to me. Look at all these individuals. They all lived in extremely different ways, with differing amounts of material possessions, and praying to different Gods. Yet, they were valuable as human beings.

Moreover, each of these cultures defined perfection differently. It was not that long ago that our own western civilization valued a plumper woman. Basically, if a lady had a little meat on her bones it showed that her father or husband had been able to supply enough food for her. She was rich. Plus, it was presumed that this healthier woman would be better suited to childbirth and the hard work that it would take to run a household.

Since I was interested in meditation, I began to notice that all cultures throughout time have taken some time for the sacred. Some pray, some contemplate, some meditate, and some make offerings to nature. Although the methods may differ substantially, these people are all doing the same basic thing. They are taking time to connect to something bigger than themselves. They are reminding themselves that the chaos of the day isn't everything. I sometimes think that this aspect is sadly lacking in our modern world.

I have slowly integrated this wisdom into the way I live my life. I looked at a variety of different ways to mediate and experimented. Eventually, I came up with my own ways that suited me and my needs. All of my tactics include some sort of meditation or visualization. I also try to meditate for ten or fifteen minutes just after lunch each day. I usually do an awareness type of meditation like a variation on counting breaths, as my main purpose is to center myself.

Another activity that has really changed the way I live my life is Reiki. In 2006, I was introduced to Reiki. I had heard of Reiki before but I had never really paid attention. I really had no clue what it was or what it did. It could have been a type of potato for all I knew.

Then, I had one of those periods of time where the universe conspired to make me listen. Within the space of a few weeks, I had two books on Reiki to review, a friend mentioned Reiki, my Dad was reading a book on it, my brother had gotten another book, and three different television shows casually mentioned Reiki as I flipped though the channels. I read the books and they really spoke to me. Within a few weeks, I had found a Master and was signed up for my first level.

At the time, I had no idea what an influence that Reiki would have on my life. As I told my husband when taking the first class, it was simply an experiment. I wasn't sure if this stuff was valid and I definitely had no forethought as to what I might do with the knowledge I might gain.

As it happens, Reiki works well on relieving physical health issues. It is also very good as part of a good stress management system. Thus, I now I tend to use Reiki to prevent flare-ups and to relieve individual symptoms.

However, I believe the greatest benefit of this healing system is that it also works on the mental, emotional and spiritual levels. In this way, Reiki looks to the actual root of any issue. You'd be shocked at how many people I treat for terminal illness, depression, or other serious life threatening conditions where the chief cause was a deeply hidden childhood trauma, anger that was left to ferment, or a disconnection between their true self and their idealized image of who they should be.

Reiki has given me a whole new way of seeing the world. Ultimately, I have come to realize that trying to impress other people only increases the likelihood that I will have another "situation". Really, by trying to be something other than my true self, I was just abusing myself. My bouts of Chronic Fatigue Syndrome and Fibromyalgia were evidence of that. My body and mind were screaming wildly trying to get my attention, trying to make me realize what I was actually doing to myself. Basically, I was trying to punish myself. Perhaps, even in some unconscious way, I was trying to commit suicide.

Since the day I started my first Reiki course, I have done sessions every day. I frequently do self healings so that I can bring up hidden issues, face them, feel them, and then release the associated pain and suffering. I have a lot of emotional baggage, so this has been a constant effort on my part for the duration.

Most days, I also do sessions on other people. I take in clients and I volunteer for a number of different Reiki healing organizations including emergency and crisis healings for a special healing unit. I have also recently founded Allies of Hope, a collaboration of Reiki practitioners, spiritual healers, and other caring individuals who wish to send loving Reiki energies, spiritual healing and/or prayers to those in need.

I find this work very rewarding. There is nothing more valuable than knowing that you relieved someone's pain and suffering when they had nowhere else to turn. I constantly get emails with updates. It's a pretty amazing feeling.

Still, probably the greatest benefit that I get from doing these sessions is that I am reminded of that even though they are ill or in pain, these people are valuable, loved individuals. Their relatives aren't emailing me saying please help my daughter with her cancer because I can't love her if she's sick. That's absolutely ridiculous. No, it is in those dire situations that people seem to rally and focus on the here and now. They couldn't care less about body size, income, or all that extraneous crap. Love and connection are their only thoughts.

So, doing Reiki for me is pretty selfish. It makes me remember to focus my energies on what is truly important in life. It also makes me aware that I am part of something bigger and greater than myself. Suddenly, being me is more of an adventure than such a burden. Maybe I can't be completely sure about my future but I want to make each moment until then count.

12 Flexibility, Unconditional Love, and Daily Life

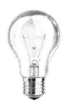

> "Dance like no one is watching. Sing like no one is listening. Love like you've never been hurt and live like it's heaven on Earth."
>
> —Mark Twain (1835-1910)

Over the past year, my attitude has been radically changing, I believe for the better. I have begun seeing myself as human. Human beings aren't perfect. They get sick. They make mistakes. They sometimes don't recognize what they have until it's taken away. I now see that Chronic Fatigue Syndrome and Fibromyalgia weren't given to me as a punishment or as proof of my impending failure. In fact, I now realize that these health issues are more likely a gift to remind me of the miracles and wonders that I do have in my life.

I sometimes wonder, would I have ever started writing my first self help book if I hadn't had the specific experiences in my life? Very likely not. I wouldn't have had any way to relate to the material I was writing. I definitely wouldn't have the passion that I have for writing without the journey that I have experienced.

Would I have opened myself up to Reiki? The old me would have written off the practice of spiritual or energy healing as mumbo jumbo. Sadly, I then would have missed out on something extremely special.

Would I have been willing to open myself up to connect with my family, friends, and perfect strangers on a deeper more honest level? I think not. I was so worried that people would judge me that I wouldn't even let my husband see the true me. I was sure that the moment he saw weakness or something he didn't agree with that he'd bolt and I would be alone. I was completely convinced that if anyone saw the real me that they couldn't help but be appalled.

Truthfully, my life is so much fuller now. I feel more comfortable being myself with my family. Although they don't always agree with my opinions or understand the intentions behind what I do, I have come to realize that their love does not depend upon these things. They love me nonetheless, as I love them.

I have always been shy, reserved, and fearful of social situations. Yet, I have noticed that I am more and more eager for the company of others. I look forward to pub nights with my husband. I actually find it enjoyable when friends join us or when my kids' friends drop by the house (so long as I'm not in my nightie). In the old days, I would have been completely overwhelmed and stressed out by these situations that I couldn't control. Now, I don't even notice any anxiety.

People are people. Some look like they have it all figured out. Trust me, they don't. They are just good actors. Some people even manage to convince themselves that they are perfect and have it all together, for a time. If you could read their thoughts though, you'd hear evidence that they are beating themselves up for what they perceive as flaws. Many people are violently jerked out of their self-made fantasies when faced with real realities of life such as adultery, divorce, death of a loved one, loss of a job, retirement, addiction, or an empty nest. Suddenly, they are forced to realize that they are human just like all the rest of us.

No one fits the ideals that our society tries to dictate to us. Few people are a natural size two. Everyone finds it difficult to juggle work and home life. Most people think they are worth more money than they are earning. No one can be all things to everyone. There are just too many possibilities to cover.

Yet, each of us is perfect in our own unique way. That part inside me that is the genuine Tami is most definitely perfect. She isn't distracted by trauma or chaos. She always sees her life as being valuable and important. She knows that she is loved and that unconditional love is the true connection between us all. She realizes that every single day is a gift, even those times that test her coping skills or make her question her worth.

It still seems a little weird to say it, but Chronic Fatigue Syndrome and Fibromyalgia have been a huge boon in my life. Ten years ago, even two years ago, that thought would never have even crossed my mind. I would have laughed hysterically at anyone who even tried to tell me otherwise. Yet, these conditions have really forced me to notice and focus on what's really important in my life. Because of these health issues, I realize that trying to impress other people is a useless exercise that just drains me of valuable energy that could be better spent elsewhere. Every day I am reminded to spend my time and energy wisely. My life experiences have helped me realize the importance of compassion, love, and contentment. If you think about it, and allow it to be, Chronic Fatigue Syndrome and Fibromyalgia can be pretty amazing gifts.

13 Summary of My Strategies

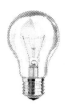

Emergency Symptom Strategies

Emergency Symptom Strategies—Legs Collapsing	
Symptoms:	• Knees joints swell and lock • Legs get weak and fatigued • Legs collapse and no longer move on their own
Coping:	• Use cane (George) to reduce mobility issues • Rest and elevate legs
Meditation:	• Relaxation Meditation and Reducing Swelling Visualization • Reiki for pain and swelling • Journaling for release of anger and frustration
Medication:	• Arthritic Rub A535 Formula on swollen knee joints

Emergency Symptom Strategies—Debilitating Fatigue	
Symptoms:	<ul><li>Intense fatigue</li><li>Horrible insomnia</li><li>Less than 4 hours sleep per night</li><li>Unrecuperative sleep</li></ul>
Coping:	<ul><li>Naps</li><li>Reduced work load</li><li>Fresh air and light exercise</li></ul>
Meditation:	<ul><li>Meditation for Relaxation and Sleep Visualization</li><li>Reiki to release toxins and induce sleep</li><li>Journaling to slow the mind and body</li></ul>
Medication:	<ul><li>Bee Pollen Extract</li></ul>

Emergency Symptom Strategies—Bowels Shutting Down	
Symptoms:	• Pain in lower abdomen • Bowels full but don't release (no constipation)
Coping:	• Warm magic bag • Eating small quantities of easy to digest foods
Meditation:	• Cleansing the System Visualization • Cleansing Reiki • Journaling to get rid of fear
Medication:	• Poria and Magnolia • Chocolate Milkshakes • Hot Blackstrap Molasses and Lemon Juice Drinks

Emergency Symptom Strategies—Monster Fibrofog	
Symptoms:	<ul><li>Confusion</li><li>Short term memory problems</li><li>Dyslexia, mixing up letters, words, opposites</li><li>Clumsiness in speech and in actions</li></ul>
Coping:	<ul><li>Lists</li><li>Calendars</li><li>Proofreading, if possible a few days later</li><li>Editors</li></ul>
Meditation:	<ul><li>Relaxation Meditation</li><li>Reiki to release synapse blockages</li><li>Journaling to release fear, frustration, and lack of control</li></ul>
Medication:	<ul><li>Ginkgo Biloba</li></ul>

Individual Symptom Strategies

Strategies for Individual Symptoms—Fatigue	
Symptoms:	• Extreme tiredness that makes the body feel heavy and the brain dim
Progression of Symptoms:	• Begins with being tired after a night of unrecuperative sleep • Sleep patterns are disrupted as a bout of insomnia begins bringing 2-3 hours of unrecuperative sleep per night • Tenseness, body aches, and grouchiness can lead to depression and body heaviness that seems impossible to break through
Coping:	• Naps • Reduced work load. • Fresh air and light exercise
Meditation:	• Meditation for Relaxation and Sleep Visualization • Reiki to release toxins and induce sleep • Journaling to slow the mind and body
Medication:	• Bee Pollen Extract • Hot Blackstrap Molasses and Lemon Juice Drinks

Strategies for Individual Symptoms—Depression	
Symptoms:	• Feelings of insecurity, dependence, and lack of value
Progression of Symptoms:	• Often starts after a few days of a debilitating bout with another symptom such as localized pain or fibrofog with a feeling of loss of control over my life • Gradually, I feel more tired, irritated, and angry • Suddenly, everything in my life seems impossible to cope with and I blame myself for not being able to fix everything and do everything that I deem I should be doing • If left unchecked, I can't make even the slightest decision for fear it is the wrong one, I can't be around others for fear of judgment, and may even feel suicidal
Coping:	• Talking to someone about my feelings • Going for a walk, getting out of the house, taking a break from the situation • Chic flick movies that allow me to cry in a safe way
Meditation:	• Awareness Meditation • Reiki to release fear and unblock feelings • Journaling to allow me to express my feelings and allow me to see that it is actually fear that is really behind the feelings
Medication:	• Chamomile Tea

Strategies for Individual Symptoms—Joint Swelling	
Symptoms:	• Joints of the knees swell creating heaviness, weakness
Progression of Symptoms:	• Knee joints swell and lock • Legs get weak and fatigued • Legs collapse and no longer move on their own
Coping:	• Use cane (George) to reduce mobility issues • Rest and elevate legs
Meditation:	• Relaxation Meditation and Reducing Swelling Visualization • Reiki for pain and swelling • Journaling for release of anger and frustration
Medication:	• Arthritic Rub A535 Formula on swollen knee joints

Strategies for Individual Symptoms—Leg Pain	
Symptoms:	• Ache that starts in the hip and spreads to the lower leg and foot
Progression of Symptoms:	• Slight aching in the hip bone (usually the left hip) • Ache turns extremely painful, more so when walking - Pain quickly moves down the leg to the foot
Coping:	• Warm magic bag on hip joint • Elevate legs • Reduce mobility
Meditation:	• Relaxation Meditation and Reducing Pain Visualization • Reiki for pain and swelling • Journaling for release of anger and frustration
Medication:	• Rub A535 Formula on hip joint

Strategies for Individual Symptoms—Back Pain	
Symptoms:	• Sharp constant pain in the center of the lower back
Progression of Symptoms:	• Slight aching in the center of the lower back • Ache turns extremely painful • Is sometimes associated with cramping and pain in intestines
Coping:	• Warm magic bag on back and on intestine area • Elevate legs so hips are above the rest of the body • Warm Epson salt baths • Eating small quantities of easy to digest foods
Meditation:	• Relaxation Meditation and Reducing Pain Visualization • Reiki for pain • Journaling for release of anger and frustration
Medication:	• Rub A535 Formula on center of lower back • Robaxacet

Strategies for Individual Symptoms—Foot Pain	
Symptoms:	• Constant ache or cramping in the arches that feels like a pebble
Progression of Symptoms:	• Funny feeling in the arch that feels like a pebble is stuck there • Ache turns painful, more irritating when walking • Pain moves up the leg
Coping:	• Massage • Soaking feet in warm water
Meditation:	• Relaxation Meditation and Reducing Pain Visualization • Reiki for pain • Journaling for release of frustration
Medication:	

Strategies for Individual Symptoms—Chest Pain	
Symptoms:	• A squeezing feeling of the front and back of the chest
Progression of Symptoms:	• The frame of the back starts to ache • There is a squeezing together feeling of the back and front parts of the chest • Panic attacks, nausea, passing out can occur
Coping:	• Talking to someone to distract me from the pain and fear • Warm magic bag on chest
Meditation:	• Relaxation Meditation and Reducing Pain Visualization • Reiki for pain and relaxation • Journaling for release of fear, anger and frustration
Medication:	• Chamomile Tea

Strategies for Individual Symptoms—Headache	
Symptoms:	• Sharp constant pain in the right temple or like a band at the back of the head
Progression of Symptoms:	• Slight headache usually in the right temple • Pain worsens and the headache expands to the back of the head like a tight band • Eyesight becomes blurry • I become extremely agitated and overwhelmed
Coping:	• Nice long relaxing bubble bath • Warm magic bag on the head (looks silly but works) • Having a nap
Meditation:	• Relaxation Meditation and Reducing Pain Visualization • Reiki for pain • Journaling for stress release and understanding of feelings
Medication:	• Advil

Strategies for Individual Symptoms—Fibrofog	
Symptoms:	• Confusion, clumsiness, dyslexia, and short term memory problems
Progression of Symptoms:	• Not completely sure of the progression • I usually first notice this symptom when I have troubles choosing between opposites or I use the wrong word in a conversation or email message
Coping:	• Lists • Calendars • Proofreading, if possible a few days later • Editors
Meditation:	• Relaxation Meditation • Reiki to release synapse blockages • Journaling to release fear, frustration, and lack of control
Medication:	• Ginkgo Biloba

Strategies for Individual Symptoms—Weight Gain	
Symptoms:	• A gradual increase in weight
Progression of Symptoms:	• Intense cravings for carbs and sugar, usually associated with a bout of other symptoms • Lack of motivation to exercise or inability to exercise due to bout of other symptoms (particularly pain) • An extra pound or two quickly turns into ten or twenty
Coping:	• Practice self soothing activities other than eating • Practice attention to hunger and fullness signs • Reduced exercise plan suited for bad bouts
Meditation:	• Relaxation and Awareness Meditation • Reiki to relieve pain and stress • Journaling to release fear, frustration, and lack of control
Medication:	• Low fat, low calorie, high nutrition cereal for carb cravings

Bout Starters

Bout Starters—Stress	
Associated Symptoms:	• Headaches, back pain, chest pain, fibrofog, weight gain
Avoidance Techniques:	• Simplify lifestyle to reduce unhealthy levels of stress • Pick and choose stressful situations only if the result will be worth it
Coping Mechanisms:	• Stay aware of fear, self defeating behavior, and anxiety levels • Stress Relief Meditation and Awareness Meditation • Journaling to release fear and anxiety • Reiki to manage stress and stay centered

Bout Starters—Lack of Sleep	
Associated Symptoms:	• Fatigue, headaches, fibrofog, weight gain
Avoidance Techniques:	• Relaxation Meditation • Fresh air
Coping Mechanisms:	• Don't stress about lack of sleep • Naps • *Sleepy Time* Tea • Journaling to release fear and anxiety • Reiki to manage fatigue and remain positive

Bout Starters—Overexertion	
Associated Symptoms:	• Fatigue, headaches, fibrofog, weight gain • Back pain
Avoidance Techniques:	• Judge activities based upon daily energy and abilities • Take breaks between tasks • Say No when it's too much
Coping Mechanisms:	• Get lots of rest and healthy foods • Meditation for Pain Relief • Journaling to release fear, anxiety, and self judgment • Reiki to manage fatigue and pain

Bout Starters—Unbalanced Routine	
Associated Symptoms:	• Fatigue, headaches, fibrofog, weight gain • Back pain
Avoidance Techniques:	• Judge activities based upon daily energy and abilities • Take breaks between tasks • Say No when it's too much
Coping Mechanisms:	• Get lots of rest and healthy foods • Meditation for Pain Relief • Journaling to release fear, anxiety, and self judgment • Reiki to manage fatigue and pain

Bout Starters—Other Illness	
Associated Symptoms:	• Fatigue, headaches, back pain
Avoidance Techniques:	• Take care of heath to reduce likelihood of getting other illnesses
Coping Mechanisms:	• Take slow days • Meditation for Relaxation • Journaling to release anxiety • Reiki to manage illness

Bout Starters—Menstruation	
Associated Symptoms:	• Fatigue, headaches, back pain
Avoidance Techniques:	• Wait until menopause
Coping Mechanisms:	• Take a slow first day • Meditation for Pain Relief of cramps • Journaling to release fear and anxiety • Reiki to manage fatigue and pain

Bout Starters—Weather Changes	
Associated Symptoms:	• Leg pain • Swelling joints • Foot pain • Back pain
Avoidance Techniques:	• Move to a climate with no weather changes
Coping Mechanisms:	• Meditation for Awareness and Pain Relief • Journaling to release fear and anxiety • Reiki to manage pain

Preventative Strategies

Preventative Strategy—Meditation	
Foundation of Strategy:	• Relaxes and centers, reminding me what's really important in life
Schedule:	• Daily after lunch • Just before bed if needed to help with sleep

Preventative Strategy—Journaling	
Foundation of Strategy:	• Lets me safely release my fears, anxieties, and anger and then reflect on the real issue
Schedule:	• Daily after breakfast • Anytime I start to really get anxious or angry

Preventative Strategy—Exercise	
Foundation of Strategy:	• Gives me more energy and stamina to get through my day
Schedule:	• Weekdays after dealing with emails and the review site • At least once a week in the afternoon: a walk in the park

Preventative Strategy—Nutrition	
Foundation of Strategy:	• Gives me more energy to get through my day
Schedule:	• Try to choose whole non-processed foods when eating • Eat until I am no longer hungry

Preventative Strategy—Reiki	
Foundation of Strategy:	• Relaxes and centers, reminding me what's really important in life
Schedule:	• Once a week while watching television

Preventative Strategy—Looking Within	
Foundation of Strategy:	• Reminding me what's really important in life and that I am a valuable person just as I am
Schedule:	• A constant work in progress

Self-Soothing Strategies

Self-Soothing Strategies

- A few deep breaths
- Meditation
- Journaling
- Reiki
- A nice warm bubble bath
- Going for a walk
- Warm Magic Bag
- Warm cup of Chamomile tea
- Lighting a candle
- Drawing/ coloring
- Talking with a friend or family member
- Any Keanu Reeves movie
- Sitting in my garden
- Reading a good book
- Chocolate

14 Marshalling Your Resources

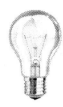

Strategy Forms

Symptoms and Strategies			
Date:			
Symptom	**Severity***	**Strategy**	**Result**

*Rate your subjective severity on a scale from 1 - 10 (minor to unbearable)

Symptoms and Strategies			
Date:			
Symptom	**Sever-ity**[*]	**Strategy**	**Result**

*Rate your subjective severity on a scale from 1 - 10 (minor to unbearable)

Symptoms and Strategies			
Date:			
Symptom	**Sever-ity***	**Strategy**	**Result**

*Rate your subjective severity on a scale from 1 - 10 (minor to unbearable)

Symptoms and Strategies			
Date:			
Symptom	**Sever-ity**[*]	**Strategy**	**Result**

[*]Rate your subjective severity on a scale from 1 - 10 (minor to unbearable)

Emergency Strategies
Symptom(s):
Coping:
Meditation:
Medication:

Emergency Strategies	
Symptom(s):	
Coping:	
Meditation:	
Medication:	

Emergency Strategies	
Symptom(s):	
Coping:	
Meditation:	
Medication:	

Emergency Strategies	
Symptom(s):	
Coping:	
Meditation:	
Medication:	

Strategies during the Worst Times

Overall Strategies:

Nutrition:

Exercise:

Meditation:

Self Discovery:

Health Care:

Particular Symptoms:

Strategies for Individual Symptoms	
Symptoms:	
Progression of Symptoms:	
Coping:	
Meditation:	
Medication:	
Notes:	

Strategies for Individual Symptoms	
Symptoms:	
Progression of Symptoms:	
Coping:	
Meditation:	
Medication:	
Notes:	

Strategies for Minor to Moderate Symptoms

Overall Strategies:

Nutrition:

Exercise:

Meditation:

Self Discovery:

Health Care:

Particular Symptoms:

Bout Starters:	
Associated Symptoms:	
Avoidance Techniques:	
Coping Mechanisms:	

Bout Starters:	
Associated Symptoms:	
Avoidance Techniques:	
Coping Mechanisms:	

Bout Starters:	
Associated Symptoms:	
Avoidance Techniques:	
Coping Mechanisms:	

Bout Starters:	
Associated Symptoms:	
Avoidance Techniques:	
Coping Mechanisms:	

Prevention Strategy:	
Foundation of Strategy:	
Schedule:	

Prevention Strategy:	
Foundation of Strategy:	
Schedule:	

Prevention Strategy:	
Foundation of Strategy:	
Schedule:	

Prevention Strategy:	
Foundation of Strategy:	
Schedule:	

Preventative Strategies	
Overall Strategies:	
Nutrition:	
Exercise:	
Meditation:	
Self Discovery:	
Health Care:	
Particular Symptoms:	

Preventative Strategies
Overall Strategies:

Nutrition:
Exercise:
Meditation:
Self Discovery:
Health Care:

Particular Symptoms:

Self Soothing Strategies:

Strategies:

Self Soothing Strategies:

Strategies:

Keeping Upbeat

Favorite Meditations, Visualizations

Inspirational Quotes

Affirmations

Fun Things You Can Still Do

Fun Things You Can Still Do

Getting Organized

Medical History	
Family History/ Risk Factors:	
Major Illnesses:	**Approximate Date:**
Operations/ Surgeries:	**Approximate Date:**

List of Medications		
Type of Medication:	**Purpose:**	**Directions:**

List of Medications		
Type of Medication:	Purpose:	Directions:

Doctor/Health Care Contacts		
Doctor:	**Specialty:**	**Contact Information:**

Special Notes:

Appointments and Procedure Schedule		
Date and Time:	**Purpose:**	**Location:**

Appointments and Procedure Schedule

Date and Time:	Purpose:	Location:

Appointments and Procedure Schedule		
Date and Time:	**Purpose:**	**Location:**

Appointments and Procedure Schedule		
Date and Time:	**Purpose:**	**Location:**

Priority List		
Most Important	**Should Do**	**Could Do**

Priority List		
Most Important	**Should Do**	**Could Do**

Priority List		
Most Important	**Should Do**	**Could Do**

Priority List		
Most Important	**Should Do**	**Could Do**

A

Medications and Supplements

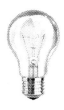

You can use this as a shopping list, try each of them and see if they help your symptoms. Always advise your medical professionals of all supplements you may be taking and any changes in diet or medication.

Advil: (ibuprophen 200mg) a.k.a. Nurofen, Nuprin, Motrin, et. al. Available at pharmacies and grocery stores.

Arthritis Rub A535: only available in Canada (Medicinal Ingredients: Methyl Salicylate 18.0%, Camphor 1.0%, Menthol 0.75%, Eucalyptus Oil 0.5%). Somewhat similar in composition to Bengay Cream as sold in the USA. http://www.viscs.com/Rub_A535.php

Bee Pollen Extract: a naturally made product available widely at health food stores. http://www.bee-health-product.com/

Blackstrap Molasses & Lemon Tea: add one tablespoon of molasses and one tablespoon of honey to 8oz boiled water. Substitute honey if molasses is not available. Sweeten to taste.

Chamomile Tea: available at any health food store or pharmacy

Epsom Salts: An Epson salt bath is known to relieve aching limbs, muscle strain and back pain. For external use only. Available at most pharmacies

Flax Seed Oil (a.k.a. Linseed Oil): produced from a blue flower in Western Canadian prairies, it is said to reduce fatigue. Available in health food stores.

Gazelle Edge Glider: a non-impact, self-powered exercise machine (see www.FitnessQuest.com)

Ginkgo Biloba: produced from trees of the same name. Available at most pharmacies. http://en.wikipedia.org/wiki/Ginkgo

Magic Bag: a bag of grain that can be heated and then applied directly to an area of pain. Provides warm, moist heat after microwaving, or cold (if stored in a freezer). Similar in composition to the Natural Pack (www.NaturalPack.com)

Magnolia Bark: Chinese herbalists have used Magnolia medicinally since the first century. Be sure to check the formulation as different parts of the plant (bark, flower, leaves) have different uses.

Poria: Poria is very widely used in Chinese herbalism. It is traditionally used as a Qi tonic to benefit the internal organs. It is a solid fungus which grows on the roots of old pine trees. It is mildly diuretic and sedative, and is considered to be highly nourishing.

Reiki: see discussion beginning on p. 45.

Robaxacet: Back Pain relief formulation mainly available in Canada. (Methocarbamol 400 mg, Acetaminophen 325 mg) http://www.backrelief.ca/

Sleepy Time Tea™: from Celestial Seasons available in most health food stores.

Vitamin B Complex: The B-vitamins are often called the "stress" vitamins. When our bodies are forced to withstand the demands of physical or emotional stress, the B-vitamins and other key nutrients are the first to be depleted.

Vitamin E: helps prevent oxidative stress by working together with a group of nutrients that prevent oxygen molecules from becoming too reactive. This group of nutrients includes vitamin C, glutathione, selenium, and vitamin B3.

B Resource Guide

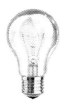

Discussion/ Support Groups

Alternative Medicine Forum
http://health.groups.yahoo.com/group/Alternative_Medicine_Forum/

CF Alliance
http://health.groups.yahoo.com/group/CFAlliance/

CFS-FM Experimental: Experimental Treatment of CFS/FM
http://health.groups.yahoo.com/group/CFSFMExperimental/

Chronic Pain Assistance
http://health.groups.yahoo.com/group/Chronic_Pain_Assistance/

Chronic Pain: Support for Chronic Pain
http://health.groups.yahoo.com/group/chronic_pain/

Cure Drive, The
http://health.groups.yahoo.com/group/The-Cure-Drive/

Fibrohugs Support Group
http://health.groups.yahoo.com/group/FibrohugsSupportGroup/

Fibro-myalgia
http://health.groups.yahoo.com/group/fibro-myalgia/

Fibromyalgia-N-Hugs
http://health.groups.yahoo.com/group/Fibromyalgia-N-Hugs/

Fibromyalgia Support Group: Fibromites Support Group
http://health.groups.yahoo.com/group/Fibromyalgia_Support_Group/

Fibromyalgia-CFS: Fibromyalgia & Chronic Fatigue Syndrome
http://health.groups.yahoo.com/group/Fibromyalgia-CFS/

Fibromyalgia Cured: Curing Fibromyalgia
http://health.groups.yahoo.com/group/fibromyalgiacured/

Immune System Health

http://health.groups.yahoo.com/group/Immune_System_Health/

RA Support: Rheumatoid Arthritis, Lupus, Fibromyalgia

http://health.groups.yahoo.com/group/RA-SUPPORT/

Women of Courage

http://health.groups.yahoo.com/group/WomenOfCourage/

Health Care, Organizations, and Agencies

All About Multiple Sclerosis: Lots of articles about the symptoms, testing procedures, and treatments as well as personal stories. http://www.mult-sclerosis.org/

American Fibromyalgia Syndrome Association: Nonprofit organization dedicated to research, education and patient advocacy for fibromyalgia syndrome (FMS) and chronic fatigue syndrome (CFS). http://www.afsafund.org/

Arthritis Society, The: Basic information on Fibromyalgia. http://www.arthritis.ca/types%20of%20arthritis/fibromyalgia/default.asp

Better Self Esteem: This site has a number of useful articles about self esteem. http://www.utexas.edu/student/cmhc/booklets/selfesteem/selfest.html

Biotech: Scientific dictionary, articles, links to scientific research and information pages for average people and professionals. http://biotech.icmb.utexas.edu/

Body Positive: Inspirational articles about healthy realistic body image. http://www.bodypositive.com/

Capita Selecta 1996: Articles summaries of articles about the immune system and Chronic Fatigue Syndrome. http://freespace.virgin.net/david.axford/mecap96.htm

CFIDS Association, The: News, brochures, and publications about Chronic Fatigue and other Immune Dysfunction Syndromes. http://www.cfids.org/

CFIDS Report, The: Links to articles and research. http://cfidsreport.com/

Co-Cure: An information exchange forum. http://www.co-cure.org/

Depression.com: Information about the symptoms, causes, and treatment of depression. http://www.depression.com/

Department of Health, Centers for Disease Control and Prevention: Information about the symptoms, diagnosis, and treatment of Chronic Fatigue Syndrome as well as support groups. http://www.cdc.gov/cfs/

Emotions Anonymous: A 12-Step program for those with recovery from difficult emotional states. http://www.emotionsanonymous.org/

Fibrant Living: Blog and podcast about living life to its fullest despite Fibromyalgia, CFS or other chronic illnesses. http://fibrantliving.com/

Fibromyalgia Network: Articles, publications, resources, and support. http://www.fmnetnews.com/

Fibromyalgia Support: popular articles about Fibromyalgia and chat room support. http://www.fibromyalgiasupport.com/

FM/CFS Canada: Research, articles, and online questions. http://fm-cfs.ca/home.html

Friends with Fibro: Information, links, and support groups. , http://www.friendswithfibro.org/

Healing Well: Books and online resources about Fibromyalgia. http://www.healingwell.com/fibro/

Illness: List of Chronic Fatigue Syndrome links. http://hsl.mcmaster.ca/tomflem/cfs.html

Internet Encyclopedia of Philosophy: Links to online philosophical articles, texts and biographies. http://www.iep.utm.edu/

Kids' Health for Parents: information on Chronic Fatigue Syndrome for parents. http://www.kidshealth.org/parent/system/ill/cfs.html

Listening to CFIDS: Writing and art of people with Chronic Fatigue and Immune Dysfunction Syndrome. http://wwcoco.com/cfids/

Living With...: A collection of information on Fibromyalgia Syndrome, Myofascial Pain Syndrome and Rheumatoid Arthritis. , http://www.livingwith.org/

Mayo Clinic: Symptoms, treatments, coping skills, and complementary medicine.
http://www.mayoclinic.com/health/fibromyalgia/DS00079

ME/CFS Medical Articles: List of medical articles.
http://freespace.virgin.net/david.axford/melist.htm

ME & FM Manual: Shows the content of the M.E. & FM Manual Newsletter. http://www.geocities.com/CapitolHill/1544/

More Self Esteem.com: Tips, articles, and books on building self esteem. http://www.more-selfesteem.com/

Myalgic Encephalomyelitis/ Chronic Fatigue Syndrome Foothold: Articles, personal experiences, and lots of other great resources.
http://notdoneliving.net/foothold/

National Association for Self-Esteem: an organization dedicated to integrity and personal/social responsibility. http://www.self-esteem-nase.org/

National Fibromyalgia Association: General information, research, alternative therapies, and coping strategies.
http://www.fmaware.org/fminfo/brochure.htm

National Mental Health Information Center: This information center contains articles and publications on all sorts of mental health issues including self esteem.
http://www.mentalhealth.samhsa.gov/publications/allpubs/SMA-3715/

Overdependence: This site has a listing of the personality traits of overdependence. It also includes online discussion and forums.
http://emoclear.com/clusters/overdependence.html

Positive Self-Esteem Reduces the Chance of Co-Dependency: Some startling statistics about violence against women. http://self-help.vocaboly.com/archives/319/positive-self-esteem-reduces-the-chance-of-co-dependency/

Psychology Self-Help Resources on the Internet: Articles, links, discussion forums for emotional health issues.
http://www.psywww.com/resource/selfhelp.htm

Self-Esteem Games: A fun site that provides games that are meant to change certain habits of thought into more healthy positive self images. http://www.selfesteemgames.mcgill.ca/games/index.htm

Support Path.com: Online chat and resources for a variety of physical realities. http://www.supportpath.com/

Women's Health Matters: Information about Chronic Fatigue Syndrome and Fibromyalgia from an environmental illness perspective. http://www.womenshealthmatters.ca/centres/environmental/chronicFatigue/index.html

Bibliography

Arenson, G. (2001). *Five Simple Steps to Emotional Healing: The Last Self-Help Book You Will Ever Need.* Wichita, KS: Fireside.

Azar LeBlanc, J. (2004). *Many Places to Many Places.* Longwood, FL: Xulan Press.

Bauman, M. (2005). *Fight Fatigue: 6 Simple Steps to Maximize Your Energy.* Mustang, OK: Tate Publishing, LLC.

Beck, M. (2007). *The Four Day Win.* New York, NY: Rodale, Inc.

Becker, H. (2007). *Unconditional Love: An Unlimited Way of Being.* Tampa, FL: White Fire Publishing.

Berger, A. and C. deSwaan. (2006). *Healing Pain: The innovative Breakthrough Plan to Overcome Your Physical Pain & Emotional Suffering.* Emmaus, PA: Rodale, Inc.

Brady, T. (2006). *The Complete Being: Finding and Loving the Real You.* Ann Arbor, MI: Loving Healing Press.

Brady, T. (2007) *Regaining Control: When Love Becomes a Prison.* Ann Arbor, MI: Loving Healing Press.

Brown, B. (2007). *I Thought It Was Just Me.* London, England: Gotham Books.

Browne, S. (1999). *The Other Side and Back: The Psychic's Guide to Our World and Beyond.* New York, NY: Dutton.

Casey, K. (2006). *All We Have is All We Need: Daily Steps Towards a Peaceful Life.* York Beach, ME: Conari Press.

Craighead, L. (2006). *The Appetite Awareness Workbook.* Oakland, CA: New Harbinger Publications, Inc.

Drury Kliment, F. (2002). *The Acid Alkaline Balance Diet.* New York: McGraw-Hill.

Finando, D. and S. Finando. (2005). *Trigger Point Therapy for Myofascial Pain.* Rochester, VT: Healing Arts Press.

Gallo, F. and H. Vincenzi. (2000). *Energy Tapping.* Oakland, CA: New Harbinger Publications, Inc.

Grabhorn, L. (2000). *Excuse Me, Your Life is Waiting.* Charlottesville, VA: Hampton Roads Publishing Company, Inc.

Guerra, B. (2005). *A Woman's Guide to Manifestation: Creating Your Reality with Conscious Intent.* San Antonio, TX: Living Life Publishing Co.

Guerra, B. (2005). *The 8 Steps to Manifestation: A Handbook/ Workbook for Conscious Creation.* San Antonio, TX: Living Life Publishing Co.

Jarrell, D. (1996). *Reiki Plus Natural Healing.* Key Largo, FL: Reiki Plus Institute.

Jeffers, S. (2005). The *Feel the Fear Guide to Lasting Love.* Santa Monica, CA: Jeffers Press.

Josefine, C. (2004). *The Spiritual Art of Being Organized.* Eureka, CA: Winter's Daughter Press.

Johnson, C. (2001). *Self-Esteem Comes in All Sizes: How to Be Happy and Healthy at Your Natural Weight.* Carlsbad, CA: Gurze Books.

Jordan, E. (2006). *The Laws of Thinking.* Manchester, CT: Foghorn Publishers.

Kaip, S. (2005). *The Woman's Workplace Survival Guide.* Medford, OR: Advantage Source.

Kersen, I. (2004). *Power is not a 4-Letter Word.* Secaucus, NJ: The Power Edge Media.

Kitabu Turner, V. (2006). *Soul To Soul: Harnessing the Power of Your Mind.* Charlottesville, VA: Hampton Roads Publishing Company, Inc.

Koven, J. (2004). *Going Deeper: How to Make Sense of Your Life When Your Life Makes No Sense.* Cathedral City, CA: Prism House Press.

Krulikowski, C. (2006). *Living a Radical Peace: Creating Life Anew.* Baltimore, MA: Publish America.

Levey, J. and M. Levey. (2006). *Luminous Mind: Meditation and Mind Fitness*. San Francisco, CA: Conari Press.

Lewis, M. (2004). *Making Right Turns in Your Relationship*. Harbour Springs, MI: Hansyd Publishing.

Maitland, A. (2000). *Master Work*. Berkley, CA: Dharma Press.

Malin, D. (2007). *Embracing Change: Transforming Life's Challenges with Courage and Grace*. New York, NY: Beaufort Books.

McCormick, B. (2001). *At Work With Thomas Edison*. Newburgh, NY: Entrepreneur Press.

McCormick, B. (2005). *Ben Franklin: America's Original Entrepreneur*. Newburgh, NY: Entrepreneur Press.

McKay, M. and C. Sutker. (2005). *The Self Esteem Guided Journal: 10-Week Program*. Oakland, CA: New Harbinger Publications, Inc.

Moland, T. (2003). *Mom Management: Managing Mom Before Everybody Else*. Calgary, AB: The Gift of Time.

Moss, R. (2007). *The Mandala of Being*. Novato, CA: New World Library.

Munseon, N. (2006). *Spiritual Lessons for My Sisters: How to Get Over the Drama and Live Your Best Life!* New York, NY: Hyperion.

Nolen- Hoeksema, S. (2006). *Eating, Drinking, Overthinking*. New York, NY: Henry Holt and Company.

Orloff, J. (2004), *Positive Energy: 10 Extraordinary Prescriptions for Transforming Fatigue, Stress & Fear into Vibrance, Strength & Love*. New York, NY: Three Rivers Press.

Pearsall, P. (2002). *Toxic Success: How to Stop Striving and Start Thriving*. Maui, HI: Inner Ocean Publishing, Inc.

Porter, C. (2001). *A Woman's Path to Wholeness: The Gift is in the Process*. Woodstock, GA: Empower Productions.

Porter, C. (2003). *The Realness of a Woman: A Journey for Seeking, Remembering & Being Who You Are*. Woodstock, GA: Empower Productions.

Post, S. and J. Neimark (2007). *Good Things Happen to Good People.* New York, NY: Random House, Inc.

Pritchard, J. and S. Lindenburger (2006). *The Warrior Mind.* New York, NY: AMACOM.

Read Hawthorn, J. (2004). *The Soul of Success: A Woman's Guide to Authentic Power.* Deerfield Beach, FL: Health Communications, Inc.

Rees, E. (2006). *S.H.A.P.E.: Finding & Fulfilling Your Unique Purpose for Life.* Grand Rapids, MI: Zondervan.

Samano, G., M. Jeffcoat, and D. Uth (2005). *I Can: Discovering the Real Truth About Change.* Winston-Salem, NC: Punch Press.

Sansone, K. (2006). *Woman First, Family Always.* Des Moines, IA: Meredith Books.

Scherer, K. and E. Bodoh. (2004). *Gratitude Works: Open Your Heart to Love.* Greendale, WI: K &E Innovations LLP.

Selak, J. and S. Overman. (2005). *You Don't Look Sick!* Binghamton, NY: The Haworth Medical Press.

Setan, S. and S. Kornblatt. (2005). *365 Energy Boosters.* York Beach, ME: Conari Press.

Shoman, M. (2004). *Living Well with Chronic Fatigue Syndrome and Fibromyalgia: What Your Doctor Doesn't Tell You...That You Need to Know.* London: Collins.

Steelsmith, L. (2005). *Natural Choices for Women's Health.* New York, NY: Three Rivers Press.

Steinfeld, J. (2006). *I've Seen a Lot of Famous People Naked, and They've Got Nothing on You!* New York, NY: AMACOM.

Stoll, W. and J. DeCourtney. (2006). *Recapture Your Health.* Boulder, CO: Sunrise Health Couch Publications.

Swift, W. (2007). *Life on Purpose: Six Passages to an Inspired Life.* Santa Rosa, CA: Elite Books.

Tavaris, C. and E. Aronson. (2007). *Mistakes Were Made (but not my Me)*. Orlando, FL: Harcourt Books.

Tulku, T. (1991). *Skillful Means*. Berkley, CA: Dharma Press.

Tulku, T. (1994). *Mastering Successful Work*. Berkley, CA: Dharma Press.

Ury, W. (2007). *The Power of a Positive No*. New York, NY: Bantam Dell.

Vad, V. (2004). *Back Rx*. New York, NY: Gotham Books.

Volkman, M. (2005). *Life Skills: Improve the Quality of Your Life with Metapsychology*. Ann Arbor, MI: Loving Healing Press.

Weldon, M. (2001). *Writing to Save Your Life: How to Honor Your Story Through Journaling*. Center City, MN: Hazelden.

Woods, J. (2006). *Soulmate or Cell-Mate*. Columbus, NC: Adawehi Press.

Wurtman, J. and N. Frusatajer Marquis (2006). *The Serotonin Power Diet*. New York: Rodale, Inc.

Wurzbacher, T. (2006). *Your Doctor Said What?: Exposing the Communication Gap*. Scottsdale, AZ: Life Success Publishing, LLC.

Index

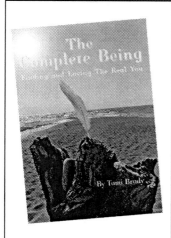

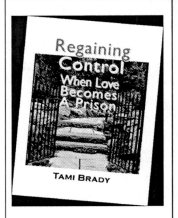

Printed in the United States
115578LV00002B/38/A